PSYCHIATRIC MENTAL HEALTH NURSING

NURSING OUTLINE SERIES

second edition

by

DORRIS B. PAYNE, Ph.D., R.N.
Assistant Dean, Graduate Program
College of Nursing
University of Florida
Gainesville, Florida

and

PATRICIA A. CLUNN, Ed.D., R.N.
Assistant Professor, Graduate Program
in Child, Adolescent and Family
Psychiatric / Mental Health Nursing
College of Nursing
University of Florida
Gainesville, Florida

MEDICAL EXAMINATION PUBLISHING COMPANY, INC.
65-36 Fresh Meadow Lane
Flushing, N.Y. 11365

PREFACE

Psychiatric nursing is a broad and complicated field of study, and the purpose of this book is to provide the nurse and student with a review, as well as an introductory, text.

Each chapter is followed by several questions which will serve as review guides. All the information necessary to answer these questions appears within the particular chapter. Suggested references, offering different views, also appear at the end of each chapter. The very end of the text contains several exercises, the answers to which are, of necessity, highly individual.

Nurses from all types of programs, students at any level, and members of other health-related professions will find this text helpful.

This book is especially helpful for students from integrated programs who are preparing for State Board Exams. It can also serve as a valuable resource for those graduates preparing for generalist certification exams.

Dorris B. Payne
Patricia A. Clunn

PSYCHIATRIC/MENTAL HEALTH NURSING
Nursing Outline Series

Second Edition

CONTENTS

PART I: INTRODUCTION

PART II: BEHAVIORS AND INTERVENTIONS

CONTENTS (Continued)

PART I: INTRODUCTION

CHAPTER 1

PAST, PRESENT AND FUTURE PRACTICE IN PSYCHIATRIC/MENTAL HEALTH NURSING

HISTORY OF PSYCHIATRIC NURSING

THE PSYCHIATRIC NURSE BEFORE 1890: Psychiatric treatment facilities developed in America much as they had in England and Western Europe. In England, one of the first asylums (Bethlem) became better known as "Bedlam" because of its uncontrolled activity and noise. By 1600, though, communities were being held liable for patient care and the government had begun funding such care.

In the late 18th century, Philippe Pinel in Belgium and William Tuke in England struck the chains from mental patients and initiated a period of humanitarian treatment. In 1796, Tuke founded the York Retreat and provided total care without restraint. No mention of nurses was made in the York reports for 50 years but then a four year training program for nurses was started and by 1908 the Retreat was training more nurses than it could employ.

In the United States, the first public hospital for mental patients was built in 1773, although mental patients had been admitted to Pennsylvania Hospital in Philadelphia for more than 20 years. Benjamin Rush, the Father of American Psychiatry, joined the Pennsylvania staff in 1783. Treatment during this period was humane and some patients were "cured". Many small hospitals were built and those who had been merely keepers of the ill became nurses of the ill.

In the middle of the 19th century, great waves of immigrants arrived in the cities. Poor, uneducated, unemployed and subjected to untold stresses, many were soon admitted to the state hospitals. By 1870, the hospitals were overcrowded, administrators began viewing patients as incurable or hopeless and the government began to pinch pennies. Once again, care became custodial and restraining.

During this time, the first Florence Nightingale school had opened at St. Thomas Hospital in London (1860). In 1873, Linda Richards, the first American psychiatric nurse, graduated from the New England Hospital for Women and Children. She organized services and educational programs in state hospitals in Illinois and helped to organize the first school to prepare nurses to care for mental patients (McLean Asylum, Waverly, Massachusetts), and Dorothea Dix, Superintendent of Women Nurses during the Civil War pioneered in reforming treatment in jails and hospitals. By 1890, another reform movement in the mental illness care system was underway.

THE PSYCHIATRIC NURSE FROM 1890-1930: Between 1890 and 1930, there was little change in the psychiatric nurse's role: long hours, low pay, poor working conditions. However, during World War I, a Central Board of Examiners established a uniform curriculum for nurses training programs in state institutions. The first textbook was published in 1920.

NURSING MENTAL AND NERVOUS DISORDERS: Clifford Beers, for three years a mental patient, wrote of his experiences in A Mind That Found Itself, published in 1908. He became interested in prevention and early detection of mental illness and founded the National Committee for Mental Hygiene. He was instrumental in initiating child guidance centers, vocational counseling and prison psychiatry.

Little changed in the psychiatric nurse's role for the next 40 years. Still mainly custodial, the care stressed physical measures. Even the so-called psychiatric procedures such as restraints or forced feedings were physical. Psychological care was defined as being kind and tolerant toward the patients and developing the right attitudes.

Psychiatry itself was still descriptive and focused upon describing and classifying behaviors. Psychiatrists were more concerned with observable "objective" symptoms or external behavior phenomena. They were not interested in any internal stimuli that might affect, determine, or control the external behaviors. Descriptive psychiatry slowly gave way to the new dynamic psychiatry. Psychiatrists became more concerned with the unconscious mental forces or the energy that they now presumed determined behavior.

Charcot, Bleuler, and Freud were some of the men who formulated the concepts of dynamic psychiatry, more concerned with the dynamics underlying the behavior than with the behavior itself.

Psychoanalysis was devised by Freud and the psyche (mind) was forever after conscious, unconscious, or somewhere in between. Freudian analysis was dependent upon a strong relationship between patient and analyst with no mediating influences. Nursing intervention was discouraged, even forbidden.

In the age of psychoanalysis, the nurse had little to contribute to the patient in the psychoanalyst's office. When analysis moved into the clinics and hospitals, the nurse became involved as a member of the treatment team.

Although nurses had become more cognizant of available knowledge and its value to nursing, they were still pessimistic about the prognosis for mental patients. Overwhelmed by the number of patients and the extreme behaviors with which they could not cope, psychiatric nurses welcomed the change that medical treatments made in both the patient and in his behavior. With somatic therapy the patient's behavior was more easily controlled and the patient became more amenable to psychotherapy. Although somatic therapy did not foster insight, in some cases (psychosurgery, for example) the patient's anxieties and feelings of inadequacy were thought to be lessened without conscious effort. In some cases, after such surgery the patient became a changed person, passive, dependent, indecisive.

These changes were not superficial changes in behavior but basic changes within the individual over which he had no control.

THE PSYCHIATRIC NURSE FROM 1930-1977: Although the somatic therapies differed in their individual procedures and their rationale, they had a common historic effect upon the psychiatric nurse.

> 1935: Insulin shock therapy
> 1935: Metrazol shock therapy
> 1936: Psychosurgery
> 1937: Electroconvulsive therapy

All the therapies required the services of skilled medical-surgical nurses. So it was that the psychiatric nurse's contribution to psychiatric treatment was built upon her manual skills in caring for the somatically treated patients.

Insulin shock involved inducing from 40-80 insulin comas over a period of 8-16 weeks. The nurse needed to monitor the depth of the coma, administer medications, and observe for relapse into a second coma.

Metrazol was used as convulsive therapy until electroshock therapy replaced it almost completely. A great disadvantage to Metrazol was that the patient was conscious until convulsions occurred and had disquieting feelings of anxiety and impending death. The nurse had to be competent in handling convulsive seizures and able to support the patient through his fears and discomfort.

In psychosurgery the nurse needed all the skills required to care for the patient before and after brain surgery. Psychosurgery was a controversial treatment because of the changes some patients experienced in personality and in cognitive functioning. Equally as controversial was the later use of psychosurgery to control recurring patterns of violent behavior.

New techniques were developed over the years and a recent study in England, (Kelly, et al.) demonstrates improvement rates ranging from 55 percent in chronic anxiety to 80 percent in depression in some 40 psychiatric patients with long-standing illnesses unresponsive to other treatment.

Somatic therapy increased the demand for improved psychological treatment for both those patients who did not respond to the somatic therapies and those whom the somatic therapies made more amenable.

As psychiatrists developed new psychotherapeutic techniques, psychiatric nurses adapted the techniques to nursing.

Psychiatrists tried to change the environment, to change the basic individual, or to help the individual function within his environment without changing either.

Psychiatric nurses were not interested in basically changing the individual. They did much to alter the environment in which the patient was confined, not just physically but by altering the communication patterns and interpersonal relationships on the ward. The psychiatric nurse was instrumental in developing milieu therapy.

The techniques most often used in psychiatric nursing evolved from communication, developmental, behavioral and psychiatric theory.

After World War II, Americans were more aware of mental illness and the psychiatric care available. They actively sought help in solving their problems and the demand for professional psychiatric personnel increased.

1946: NATIONAL MENTAL HEALTH ACT: The first broad-based mental health act brought patients into the mainstream and authorized the construction of the National Institutes of Mental Health and a program for:

1. Training professional psychiatric personnel
2. Supporting psychiatric research
3. Aiding the development of mental health programs at the state level

Psychiatric nursing was one of the four specified professions. Collegiate programs developed at both the baccalaureate and graduate levels.

The psychiatric nurse did not become a member of the treatment team until social psychiatrists and psychologists developed treatment techniques for psychotic patients. Later concepts of Community Mental Health treatment changed the role to that of full member on the multidisciplinary team.

In the 1950's, Paplau's classic book: Interpersonal Relations in Nursing provided a framework for psychiatric nursing. Schools of nursing were now required to offer courses in psychiatric nursing for purposes of accreditation. Preparation of the clinical specialist moved into graduate school and the first doctoral program in psychiatric nursing was offered at Boston University in 1960.

Traditional nursing had stressed emotional noninvolvement between patient and nurse. Many disagreements arose between the followers of "self" and the followers of "noninvolvement". Those nurses who knew that their roles were clearly defined and did not include becoming personally involved with patients thought such involvement extremely "unprofessional". They viewed their relationships with patients as business transactions involving communication patterns similar to any other impersonal interaction. They had learned specific behaviors and nursing procedures to facilitate their patient care activities and their own individuality was not considered as either important or as affecting those activities.

Those nurses who felt that they, as individuals, could contribute their own unique qualities to the nurse-patient relationship knew that involvement was unavoidable. They viewed their personal strengths and weaknesses as tools to be used in facilitating patient care. Of course, any relationship is affected by the personalities and behaviors of the individuals involved. The nurse-patient relationship is no different. The choice was never actually between use of "self" and "non-involvement". The choice was between the conscious use of self and the unconscious use of self.

Today most nursing students learn the difference between the conscious use of self in a therapeutic relationship and the emotional involvement occurring in a social relationship. The therapeutic relationship involves purposeful interaction between two individuals in which one--the nurse--is concerned with actions and behaviors that will help the other--the patient--improve. Nurses involved in therapeutic relationships are aware of their feelings and actions, of why they are doing whatever they are doing and how they can best utilize their feelings and actions to help the patient. Nurses, being human, cannot always change their feelings about individuals but they can recognize, face, and use those feelings in giving therapeutic care.

A social relationship does not involve purposeful activity or responsibility on the part of one-the nurse-to ensure help to the other-the patient. Becoming emotionally involved with a patient without recognizing the feelings and actions of both parties can develop into a social transaction in which both members are seeking to satisfy their own needs. On the other hand, the "non-involvement" approach can also become a social relationship in which the nurse may recognize, but not face, feelings and actions which affect the interaction. This type of social relationship satisfies neither party's needs and is impersonal on the "Hello, how are you, I'm fine" level. A social relationship, whether personal or impersonal, is not a helping relationship and has very little place in professional nursing.

Research at the graduate level helped test and evaluate the new techniques. Integration of psychiatric nursing concepts at the baccalaureate level theoretically prepared all graduate nurses to meet patients' psychological needs.

As the demand for psychiatric services outdistanced the supply, social psychiatry attempted to fill the void. Social psychiatry emphasized the impact of environmental influences and of social groups upon individuals not only as cause but also in prevention and treatment. The social psychiatrists developed the therapeutic community concept.

1953: MAXWELL JONES' "THE THERAPEUTIC COMMUNITY" PUBLISHED: Therapeutic communities became the preferred solution to the shortage of personnel. State and federal mental hospitals organized wards as "communities" in which patients could function in relationship to each other and to the community.

Such communities involved long-term patients in their own care instead of treating them as incompetents and fostering greater dependency. Trust replaced controls, self-direction replaced regimentation and individual dignity and desires replaced depersonalizing rituals. The patient became an active participant in his own care and in developing the social group with which he could identify. The patients were involved in the day-to-day problems of their own communities.

They helped resolve problems, plan activities, develop necessary rules and regulations. They had as much control as possible over their own personal activities. Interpersonal relationships were the foci of treatment. Patients became increasingly aware of their own behaviors within the group, of how their behaviors affected their interactions, and of how the interactions affected their self-esteem. Relationships within a social group helped patients identify problem areas and recognize "trouble before it came" thus increasing independence and decreasing the need for external controls. They learned to modify unacceptable behavior, perhaps to change long-standing non-productive attitudes and beliefs.

As new treatments were introduced, psychiatric nurses had to change from a medical to a psychiatric orientation. Unfamiliar with such social therapy techniques as halfway houses, day and night hospitals, and mental health clinics, nurses were as overwhelmed and depressed as they had been in the custodial care days.

Even those nurses who developed skills in the social milieu approaches found they had problems convincing other members of the psychiatric team that nurses had something to contribute and the team needed them. This situation still exists in many areas of the United States.

The clinical specialist developed a role as geriatric specialist, family therapist, private practitioner. She worked with children and adolescents, in hospitals and in the community. She worked in crisis intervention and in long-term care; with the mentally retarded, the substance abuser, the sexually deviant.

The theory and concepts of psychiatric nursing care and the psychiatric nurse's attitude towards patients have influenced all areas of nursing.

As the psychiatric nurse becomes more involved in crisis care (intervention on a short-term basis to avoid hospitalization and handle an immediate problem), family therapy (involvement of all family members concerned in treatment of the "patient" in the family), transactional analysis (contract between two equals to identify such basic needs as excitement, recognition, "strokes" and structure and to restructure the client's ego states), newer therapeutic techniques (encounter groups, gestalt therapy, reality therapy, sex therapy, behavior therapy, poetry therapy), more of the psychiatric nursing philosophy will be adopted by other members of the nursing profession.

As nurses move into the community with patients they will learn to value more and more the psychiatric nurse's attitude toward patient and toward self.

Psychiatric nursing has had and will have a profound historic effect upon all of nursing.

LEGAL ASPECTS OF COMMUNITY NURSING

Legal control over a profession is based in the police power of the State to protect its citizens from incompetent or fraudulent practitioners. Each state has a Nurse Practice Act which defines nursing and the responsibilities, functions and education of the profession in the individual states. Each state also has a State Board of Nursing whose members are responsible for administering the Act. Many states are revising their nurse practice acts in the wake of the recent movement toward practitioner skills and independent practice. Nurses practice - legally - within the scope of the rights and liabilities afforded by the Act in the state of practice, not the state of original licensure. Much of the law is concerned with traditional functions of nursing, especially the one dependent function: execution of physician's orders concerning treatments and medications.

As the independent functions of nurses are being emphasized more and more, the practice acts are being reviewed and revised to control them. The independent functions are:

1. Execution of nursing procedures
2. Observation and nursing diagnosis
3. Supervision of patients
4. Direction and education for physical and mental care
5. Accurate recording, reporting and evaluation of patient care
6. Supervision of other health care workers

It is in the area of independent function that the legal definitions are the most ambiguous. The ANA standards are far more precise than the law (see Appendix F) in defining responsibilities.

Legal responsibilities of nonmedical therapists have not yet been tested, and therefore, have not been well defined. The nurse involved in therapy in community centers needs to be fully cognizant of the laws of her state and to have legal advice to help her determine just where she stands, and what her responsibilities are. And she needs to carry malpractice insurance.

Theoretically, if the nurse is considered to be an employee of the psychiatrist, or works under his supervision, she is an agent of the psychiatrist and he is responsible for her work.

However, every professional practitioner has certain legal duties of care. If these duties are violated, malpractice exists. Most malpractice claims are tried under the law of negligent tort. And under the law every one is responsible for his own torts. So the nurse is responsible and can be held responsible in malpractice claims.

A tort is a wrong committed by one party involving injury to another. It is a legal wrong that is redressable in a civil rather than a criminal proceeding.

Under the law of negligent tort the plaintiff must show:

1. That a legal duty of care existed
2. The nurse performed the duty negligently
3. As a result the plaintiff accrued damages
4. The damages were substantial

Proving the claim is often difficult even though the principle of "res ipso loquitor" (the fact speaks for itself) is used. Although originally used as an inference of negligence, or as circumstantial evidence, the principle has been more often used in recent years as a presumption of negligence and the burden of proof shifts from the plaintiff to the defendant.

Basic to all malpractice is the "legal duty of care". A legal duty can be defined by:

1. Statute law (legislative)
2. Case law ("common sense" - case decisions)

Nurses have traditionally been protected by the rule of "respondeat superior" under which the employer was liable for a tort committed by an employee. This rule is not applicable for an independent contractor. As an independent practitioner, however, she does need to be conversant with the laws regarding contracts: who can legally enter into a contract; how contracts operate; the formation of contracts and how they are enforced. As more and more nurses enter into contracts, there will be an increase in suits for breach of contract, for failure to provide service, for providing inadequate or inappropriate service.

Although rarely sued for malpractice in the past, the danger of such suits has been increasing. Greater emphasis is being placed on the rights of patients (see Appendix E), especially the basic right to treatment, right to refuse treatment and right to discontinue treatment.

Psychiatric treatment changes as society changes and reflects the changing viewpoints. Diagnoses have sometimes been used as a controlling mechanism by society and sometimes as a freeing mechanism. As the attitudes toward homosexuality have changed, the APA removed homosexuality as a disease in the Diagnostic Nomenclature (see Appendix C), thereby removing previous stigma.

The nurse in the community may find herself involved in problems of divorce, involuntary admission to inpatient units, family problems involving children or adolescents, suicide, wills, drug reactions.

Accurate records will not, in themselves, absolve a defendant in a malpractice claim, but they can help. Without accurate records, many problems may not be resolvable. For instance:

1. A patient on MAO inhibitor has had precautions explained to him. He has an Italian dinner, complete with cheese and chianti. He

goes into hypertensive crisis and dies. Family sues because they were not informed and he wasn't either.

If the nurse has kept an accurate record, including the incident recounting the explanation of side effects, a claim will not be lost by the nurse, psychiatrist, or other defendant. If there is no record available, they may have a problem.

2. A child of 15 is subjected to a somatic treatment she doesn't wish to have, because her parents signed the consent form and she had no legal redress. When she reaches 18, she can file a claim for past intrusions of privacy, try the claim as an intentional tort - that is, she was deliberately handled injuriously.

A nurse may be called as a witness in any type of suit involving a patient. There is as yet no "privileged communication" between nurse and patient. A nurse who allows patients to talk about situations or actions that are irrelevant to care, and may be embarrassing if made public, is asking for problems. On a witness stand, if the irrelevant matter is a matter of importance and direct questions are asked, the nurse may be faced with such options as:

1. Relate the information and humiliate or hurt the patient
2. Lie and face possible perjury charges
3. Refuse to answer and face contempt charges

Those options are not too appealing. A community mental health nurse tries to focus upon prevention in the center and might try prevention in this case. Don't collect more information than is necessary, and if the patient insists upon telling her most personal past actions, the nurse can try "tuning-out" or tell the patient to speak to the psychiatrist who does have privileged communications.

Those options may not be appealing either, but if they can save the patient from more trauma, they are worth considering. The wrong kind of information, aired in court, can be devastating in divorce or custody suits. If the information isn't relevant to the patient's care, it doesn't need to be collected.

Two of the functions of a community mental health center are consultation and research. There are possible pitfalls here, also. In consultation, if the consultee acts upon a consultant's "advice" and error occurs, the consultant may be sued.

In doing research, it is necessary to obtain informed consent from the patient for any action taken, and to guard the patient's privacy. Communications may not be privileged but any breach of confidentiality can result in claims. Revealing any information damaging to the patient may be considered libelous.

Patients are capable of manipulating psychiatric staff into "compromising" situations. Participation in nude marathon groups, sex therapy, even on a one-to-one basis can result in false claims. This is more apt to happen to a man than a woman, but it does happen to

women. A woman's greatest danger might well arise with adolescents or lesbians.

There are many possible claims against a nurse whose legal duty of
care is not clearly defined. To avoid such claims a nurse should:

1. Know the laws of the state
2. Have a lawyer
3. Keep accurate and concise records
4. Use "common sense"
5. Refrain from collecting unnecessary information from patients
6. Maintain confidentiality of information collected at all times
7. If involved in too many claims, as the man said, "see a
    psychiatrist"

FUTURE OF COMMUNITY MENTAL HEALTH NURSING

As far back as the 12th century, the people of Gheel, Belgium cared
for the mentally ill in their homes on an "outpatient" basis. The patients were not relatives, but the Gheel residents provided foster
homes and work programs for them.

In the Dark Ages, the demons were exorcised by visits to the homes
of those bewitched, another form of taking the treatment to the
patient!

These activities may be viewed as early forms of community nursing
by stretching a point.

It was not until the 20th century that the actual concept of "mental
health" began in 1908 when Clifford Beers' account of his experiences
as a patient was published. At the same time, Adolf Meyer advocated
a plan for community mental health care. In the early twenties, the
first child psychiatric clinics were established by William Healy. The
treatment team included psychiatrist, psychologist and social worker.
Nurses were not included, and this pattern still prevails in many child
psychiatric units.

Military psychiatry showed that community mental health was a practical and workable idea. After World War II, the military's use of
group therapy, of staff recruited from the area, and of nonmedical
therapists, gave a push to the community mental health program.
Nurses had served as more than medicine nurses and doctor's help-
ers in the military, and continued to function in the community in a
limited way.

With the advent of the community mental health centers in the 1960's,
the community mental health nurse began coming into her own.

The nurse has progressed from a custodian to a medical nurse during
somatic therapy to a subsidiary member of the mental health team.
The nurse has now attained full and equal status with other members
of the team who formerly "outranked" her.

In the community mental health center the nurse has become a therapist competent in crisis intervention, and capable of functioning with the inpatient, the outpatient or the partially hospitalized. The nurse has become versed in most of the psychosocial therapies.

The nurse practiced milieu therapy long before it was fashionable or known as milieu therapy. The nurse is now competent in handling groups or families as well as one-to-one relationships.

The community mental health nurse has come a long way since 1960. What is left to accomplish?

More and more certification for specialized practice will be an issue. If the profession does not itself control the process (as it is in the process of doing now) the federal government will. Governmental control will be especially apparent when third-party payments are available for clinical nurse specialists and independent practice increases. Psychiatric nurses, always in the vanguard of change, will continue to lead nursing in this area of private practice and certification.

Mental status exams (see Appendix D) are now part of the nurse's responsibilities. In the future, she will research and develop assessment instruments for neurological examinations and ego assessments that nurses in other clinical areas may also utilize. Research and evaluation of clinical practice will help to develop nursing theory and to improve the image of nursing.

The community itself will have much to say about its own needs and its own wants. The nurse will be in the community more and more and in the Center less. The nurse will function not only in homes, but will take therapeutic intervention into industry and school, airports - perhaps even space.

Emphasis will be on maintaining the actual physical environment, on crisis intervention, on the young and on the old. The dynamic psychiatry of old will cease to be the basis for "dynamic" nursing. Freud will give way to Piaget, the id desires will be less important than cognitive functioning. Reality therapy will be universally used.

Community mental health will reflect, but probably not influence, the changing community and family structures.

Communes, rural villages, and urban ghettoes will all be the nurse's work area. It may well be in the area of occupational or industrial therapies that the nurse will have the most influence. Absenteeism, alcoholism, growing drug addiction, boredom and apathy - industry is one large crisis waiting to happen.

When the working people suffer from Future Shock and have crises precipitated by social pressures and internal emptiness, the nurse will be there to intervene.

Mental health care has been available to the rich and the poor, the psychotic or neurotic, old or young. Soon, with Federal financing, such care will be available to the "well". And the nurse will be there to intervene before problems occur.

The nurse may well become the primary provider of therapeutic care in the community. There are not enough psychiatrists to direct all the community care centers. The nurse is ready and prepared to step in and assume a greater part of the care. The role will be there to define in whatever way desired.

There have supposedly been three revolutions in psychiatry: Freud, somatic therapy, and community mental health. The fourth revolution will occur when mental health nursing care supplants psychodynamics as the guiding force in community mental health centers.

At least that's one version of the future!

REVIEW QUESTIONS

1. What was Gheel?
2. When did community mental health nursing really begin?
3. What are some of the problems the nurse may face in the future in the community?
4. Why will industrial nursing be important?
5. What will be the fourth revolution?
6. Is the psychiatric nurse a late addition to the nursing profession in America?
7. What skills did a psychiatric nurse need in the age of custodial care?
8. How do the skills needed for the social therapists differ from the skills needed for the somatic therapies?
9. Are psychiatric nursing techniques today applicable to other areas of nursing? If so, how? If not, why not?
10. What is a tort?
11. Who is legally responsible for a tort claim against a nurse?
12. How is a nurse's legal duty of care in a community mental health center defined?
13. What has to be proven in a case of negligent tort? Who has to prove it?
14. What is case law?
15. What sort of situations can lead to claims against a nurse?
16. What precautions can be taken to prevent such claims?

SUGGESTED REFERENCES

1. Bailey, H.: Nursing Mental and Nervous Diseases, The Mac millan Co., New York, 1970

2. Barber, J.B.: Psychosurgery; Viewpoint of a black neuro-surgeon, Urban Health IV:22-23/48, Oct., 1975

3. Beers, C.: A Mind That Found Itself, Longmans, Green, New York, 1908

4. Bernzweig, E.P.: Nurse's Liability for Malpractice: A Programmed Course, McGraw Hill Book Co., New York, 1969

5. Claudwell, T. and Vidaner, R.: Mental health services in the total health system, Hosp Community Psychi XXIII:200-203, July, 1972

6. Corsini, R. (Ed.): Current Psychotherapies, F. E. Peacock Publishers, Inc., Itasca, Ill., 1973

7. Creighton, H.: Law Every Nurse Should Know, W.B. Saunders, Philadelphia, 1970

8. Daly, R.W., et al.: Three views of the "Third psychiatric revolution", International J Psychi X:31-51, Sept., 1972

9. Eaton, M.T., Jr. and Peterson, M.H.: Psychiatry, Medical Examination Publishing Co., Inc., New York, 1969

10. Gibson, R.W.: Can mental health be included in the Health Maintenance Organization? Am J Psychi 128:919-926, 1972

11. Grover, E. and Gormley, E.: A study of psychiatric walk-in clinic in a general hospital, Hosp Progress LIII:70-72, Nov., 1972

12. Henderson, N.: Nursing via satellite, Can Nurse LXXII:30-33, 1976

13. Jones, M.: The Therapeutic Community, Basic Books, New York, 1953

14. Kalkman, M.: New Dimensions in Mental Health - Psychiatric Nursing, McGraw Hill, New York, 1974

15. Kelly, D., et al.: Stereotactic limbic leucotomy, Br J Psychi CXXIII:141-148, 1973

16. Leedy, J.J.: Poetry Therapy, J.B. Lippincott, Philadelphia, 1969

17. London, P.: Behavior Control, Harper and Row, New York, 1969

18. Masserman, J.H.: Theory and Therapy in Dynamic Psychiatry, Jason Aronson, New York, 1973

19. Meninger, K.: Whatever Became of Sin, Hawthorn Books, Inc., New York, 1973

20. Menninger, W.C. and Leaf, M.: You and Psychiatry, Charles Scribner & Sons, New York, 1958

21. Miller, C.L.: Nurses and the Law, Interstate Printers & Publishers, Inc., Danville, Ill., 1970

22. Moreau, D., et al.: Role of a nurse on a psychiatric consultation service, Can Psychi Assoc J XIX:453-456, 1974

23. Murchison, I. and Nichols, T.S.: Legal Foundations of Nursing Practice, The Macmillan Co., New York, 1970

24. Nelson, J. and Schilke, D.A.: The evolution of psychiatric liaison nursing, Perspectives in Psychi Care XIV:60-65, 1976

25. Palmer, I.S.: The role of history in the preparation of nurse leadership, Nursing Forum XV:117-164, 1976

26. Peplau, H.: Interpersonal Relations in Nursing, G.P. Putnam & Sons, New York, 1952

27. Piedmont, E.B. and Downey, K.J.: Revolutions in psychiatry, or the emperor's new clothes, International J Social Psychi XVII:111-121, Spring, 1971

28. Ramshorn, M.: The major thrust in American psychiatry: past, present, future, Perspectives in Psychi Care IX:44-147, 1971

29. Robinson, L.: Psychiatric Nursing as a Human Experience, W.B. Saunders Co., Philadelphia, 1972

30. Robitscher, J.: Child psychiatry and the law, Behavior Pathology of Childhood and Adolescence, Basic Books, New York, 422-438, 1973

31. Rutledge, K.A.: The professional nurse as a primary therapist; background, perspectives and opinion, J Operational Psychi V:76-86, 1974

32. Shepard, M.: A Psychiatrist's Head, Dell Publishing Co., Inc., New York, 1972

33. Shepard, M. and Lee, M.: Games Analysts Play, G.P. Putnam & Sons, New York, 1970

34. Sheridan, B.: New malpractice peril for every doctor: the battered child, Med Economics 33-46, Nov., 1976

35. Springer, E.W.: Nursing and the Law, Health Law Center, Aspen Systems Corp., Pittsburgh, 1970

36. Stone, I.: The Passions of the Mind, Doubleday, New York, 1970

37. Strauss, A., et al.: Psychiatric Ideologies and Institutions, Collier-Macmillan, Ltd., The Free Press of Glencoe, London, 1964

38. Wilhelm, Y.: A look at psychiatric commitment, Perspectives in Psychi Care IX:49-51, 1971

39. Wise, T.: Utilization of a nurse-consultant in teaching liaison psychiatry, J Med Education XLIX:1067-1068, 1974

40. Worth, B.: Reflections of psychiatric nurse patient, <u>Perspectives in Psychi Nursing</u> VII:73-75, July, 1969

CHAPTER 2

PSYCHODYNAMICS

Thoughts, impulses, and ideas are theoretically charged with emotions called psychic energy. "Psychodynamics" refers to a description or explanation of how the psychic energy is displayed or used during adaptive situations. Such dynamics influence behavior and, if correctly identified, can be used to predict behavior.

Psychodynamic nursing is based upon certain premises, adapted from dynamic psychiatry:

1. All behavior has meaning
2. All behavior can be understood
3. An individual does not always recognize his own behavior or the reasons for his behavior
4. Any behavior can be changed
5. An individual has the right to change or not to change, as he chooses - to move closer to health or to illness
6. People have a tendency to move toward health and away from illness

Thoughts, impulses and ideas originate in the mind. The mind has levels of consciousness:

1. Conscious: Awake and aware of both self and environment
2. Preconscious: Half-remembered data that can be easily brought to consciousness
3. Sub-conscious: Partly repressed data that can be brought to conscious level under some circumstances
4. Unconscious: Deeply repressed throughts, impulses, and other data essentially unavailable to the conscious mind

The mind also has structures:

1. The Id: Most primitive, instinctual selfish part of the personality. Operates on the pleasure principle and exists only in the present. Its chief function is to supply energy and creative potential to the personality. Unconscious level.
2. The Ego: The self, personal identity. Operates on the reality principle. Most logical, rational, adult part of the personality. Primary function of ego is to control the Id and the Superego, to modify them and adapt to the environment. Ego integrates the various parts of the personality and also the mental processes. Provides the thought processes and the control necessary to turn creative energy of Id into productive creativity. Represses unconscious data not wanted in the conscious. Primarily conscious.
3. The Superego: The conscience, the values, morals, and ideals acquired from parents and other outside influences. Primary function is to control instincts and assimilate the cultural values.

May sometimes fight the ego as well as the Id. Primarily unconscious.

The psychic structures of the mind have certain modes of action called mechanisms. Unconscious data not wanted in consciousness is repressed by the ego as soon as the unwanted data becomes known to consciousness. The actions involved in the repression constitute a mechanism and serve to defend the ego against anxiety, guilt, or shame arising from a conflict with Id impulses. Such mechanisms help the individual cope with feelings and situations which cannot be dealt with on a more conscious level at that time. Some mechanisms, such as compensation, sublimation, identification, can be productive and positive. Some mechanisms, such as denial, conversion, projection, can be self-defeating and negative. Whether positive or negative, productive or nonproductive, defense mechanisms do enable the individual to cope with the otherwise unmanageable events of life.

NEEDS

A need is a condition within the individual that requires action. Needs are descriptive and cause discomfort, forcing the individual to do something about the need. Needs may be internal or external in focus although all needs are felt only within the individual. Needs may arise from:

1. Internal metabolic processes (the need for sleep, for food, for water): these needs are universal, yet highly individual.
2. External environmental processes (the need for shelter, for body covering, for physical protection): these needs are also universal but vary more with the individual.
3. Internal environmental processes (the need for love, for discovery, for self-fulfillment): these needs are universal within cultures and highly individual.
4. Symbolic processes (the need for religion, for institutions, for groups): these needs are universal but vary in emphasis within cultures and eras - as do the symbols themselves (cross and ankh, wedding ring and "gay" jewelry, long hair and crew cuts).

Needs can be classified by levels:

1. Physiologic (hunger)
2. Safety (avoiding harm)
3. Love (both giving and receiving)
4. Esteem (self-respect and respect of others)
5. Self-actualization (achieve one's full potential) (Maslow)

If basic or lower level needs are not met, satisfaction of higher level needs is postponed. An individual may face danger to obtain food but rarely stops to make love when his life is threatened. Self-esteem suffers when love needs are not met and self-actualization is not possible without self-respect. So each level both builds upon and includes the preceding lower levels.

Sometimes needs are in conflict. How an individual handles such conflict depends upon his own responses, his cultural norms, the incompatible feelings and reactions of both the individual and his culture. Conflicts may be of different types:

1. Two pleasurable needs can be gratified. Example: A girl can marry a man who builds her self-esteem or a man who loves her.
2. A pleasurable need can be gratified but another need cannot be gratified. Example: Individual wins an airlines contest prize of two weeks in Hawaii, but he is afraid of flying.
3. Two needs, neither of which can be gratified without frustrating the other, threaten an individual. Example: Husband ridicules wife for being fat. She can continue to enjoy eating and lose his love, or she can keep his love by not eating.

The end results of conflict may be tension and stress of various strength and various duration, and a loss of response choices. If the stress becomes too great for an individual who is goal-directed, he may not be able to keep his goal in sight and satisfy his needs.

If the stress is beyond the individual's tolerance limit, he will become frustrated and no longer goal-directed. He may respond with aggression, regression, or apathy, none of which are goal-directed, but all of which reduce the tension.

Stress and frustration influence behavior. Needs arise from a state of tension and are the basis of overt and covert behavior.

BEHAVIOR

Behavior describes an individual's response to stimulus.
Behavior may be:

1. Reflex action: immediate response to external stimulus (knee jerk, military salute, conditional response to hard hats or long hair)
2. Goal-directed: attainment of a specific goal to satisfy an internal need (marriage, writing a book, going to school)
3. Nonproductive: frustration in attaining goal or no specific goal to satisfy an internal need (two men have needs for marriage and family - one moves to the YMCA, the other is rejected by his lover and kills her)

Anxiety may greatly affect behavior. When anxiety increases above an individual's tolerance level, awareness is reduced, energy is spent on defense, memory and learning ability are decreased.

Nurses deal primarily with the patient's total behavior in their professional work. Nursing care is based upon behavior.

Behavior is influenced by the entire individual. Example: Patient is excitable and hyperactive, has an electrolyte imbalance. Care is based on both the observable behavior and the physiological behavior, on the total behavior.

Behavior is influenced by an individual's energy level at a given time. Example: Patient may be apathetic because of little energy, and not just withdrawn. May need rest rather than activities and/or group participation.

All behavior has meaning. Behavior occurs to satisfy needs by keeping something, gaining something, or losing something. Example: A patient alone for three days in a two-bed room may try to maintain his privacy by abusing anyone who enters his room; may try to gain companionship by reminding every nurse that the second bed is still empty; may try to get rid of his "problem" by asking advice of everyone. All the behaviors have meaning and purpose.

Behavior is caused. Example: A patient's temperature spikes; he complains of a headache; he refuses to see his visitors. All may be related but each one has a cause.

Behavior at a specific moment is the best behavior the individual can show. Example: One person may react with anger, another with tears, a third with a good humored laugh. Each one is coping the best he can at that moment.

Behavior reflects not what has happened but what the individual has perceived as happening. Example: An individual will react and behave differently if he perceives a gesture as being helpful than he would if he perceived the gesture as being dangerous.

Behavior reflects needs satisfied and will not change unless needs are satisfied. Example: A patient will not cooperate in therapy if he has missed two meals and is hungry.

Behavior can be changed, but the individual involved must change it himself. Example: Nothing a nurse can do will make a patient join a group or behave more appropriately if he doesn't want to. But she can provide a facilitating environment and reinforce his positive constructive behaviors.

Any behavior or aspect of behavior has implications for nursing care. Nursing care is actually involved with nothing except behavior.

DEFENSE MECHANISMS

There are many defense mechanisms. Sometimes a variety of mechanisms are used in one situation. Sometimes an individual tries to use the same mechanisms in every situation. Defense mechanisms (except suppression) are unconscious and "protect" the ego. Some of the more common mechanisms are:

1. Displacement: Feelings are distorted, separated from the original object, and discharged toward a substitute object. Example: Father, embarrassed in public meeting by his boss, comes home and ridicules his son in front of the son's friends.
2. Denial: Painful or anxiety-inducing aspects of reality are blocked out. Example: Mother has been told her child is severely re-

tarded; she still plans ahead for college because Uncle Joe was slow as a child, too - and he's a Ph.D.

3. Compensation: A real or imagined inadequacy is alleviated by substituting another goal to maintain own self-respect and gain others' approval. Example: The frightened boy who becomes a daredevil auto racer.

4. Regression: Behavior patterns characteristic of an earlier period are displayed. Example: A five-year-old is hospitalized and begins to suck his thumb.

5. Conversion: Feelings become unbearable and are rechanneled somatically. Example: Man wants to beat a friend but can't close his hand into a fist, fingers will not curve.

6. Projection: Undesirable feelings are attributed to others. Example: Archie Bunker calling his wife a "dingbat".

7. Rationalization: Unacceptable feeling responses are justified or excused with logical reasons. Example: A girl cannot afford a dress she likes and says "It made me look too fat anyway".

8. Sublimation: Unacceptable impulses are discharged indirectly in constructive activities. Example: Children make mud pies or fingerpaint instead of smearing.

9. Reaction formation: Unresolved conflicts between feelings or impulses alleviated by reinforcing one and repressing the other. Example: Hostile woman who gushes sweetness and "loves" everyone.

10. Identification: Feelings, qualities, attributes of someone admired are imitated until they become an actual part of the individual. Example: Boy who imitates father and becomes very much like his father.

11. Isolation: Certain feelings, ideas, are set apart from others; the emotional and intellectual content are separated. Example: Nurse stresses "humanistic" hospital care, but refuses to let parents stay with their children.

12. Introjection: Feelings, values, attitudes of another assimilated into own ego or superego. Example: Small child whose parents literally become a part of him.

13. Undoing: Actions are negated by other actions. Example: Man proposes on a romantic night, does not again mention marriage and introduces girl to his best friend.

14. Condensation: A group of ideas is expressed by a single word and the single word is reacted to with all the emotions associated with the group of ideas. Example: Any four letter word synonymous with sex.

15. Repression: Unwanted feelings are kept out of awareness. Example: Girl is jealous of her brother but has never been aware of it.

16. Suppression: Unwanted feelings are consciously kept out of awareness. Example: Scarlet O'Hara's "I'll think about that tomorrow".

Transference is another unconscious mechanism which also exists outside the therapy situation, occuring in all significant relationships. In psychoanalytic terms the patient projects his feelings, thoughts, and wishes onto the therapist and the person is reacted to as if he were someone from the past. Behaviors that might have been appropriate when small are inappropriate in the patient. In a postive transference, the nurse is idolized. In a negative transference, the nurse becomes "bad". Neither feeling has a reality basis.

Countertransference occurs when the therapist identifies with the patient and reacts as if to someone from the past. Such situations are sometimes termed personality clashes.

All strong emotional reactions are not transference or countertransference. Poor nursing care remains poor nursing care and the patients may object or complain. They are not having a problem with transference. Transference can be used therapeutically to help the patient work through his problems but when the nursing care is poor, improve the care and don't label the patient's anger or hostility as transference.

Defense mechanisms aid in solving problems and in adjusting to reality. Failure to adjust efficiently can threaten the very life, and individuals try to adjust as effectively as possible. As environmental conditions change, individuals vary their responses to the change. Problems can be solved by adopting new responses, by changing the environment, or by modifying needs.

CHANGE, STRESS AND ADAPTATION

Stress is described as the "rate of wear and tear on the body" or "the sum of nonspecific changes caused by function or damage" (Selye, p. 274). Stress is any factor that requires a response or change in the individual; stressors can be due to physical, chemical, microbiological, physiological, developmental and/or emotional factors. The General Adaptation Syndrome (GAS) holds that both positive and negative changes can be stressors; winning a game of tennis can cause as much an increase in the general adaptation response as painfully stubbing one's toe or having a cold.

The nonspecific bodily reactions to stress are best described by Cannon's "fight or flight" reaction: elevated blood pressure, restriction of bodily fluids, increased muscle activity, pupillometric changes, all mediated by hormonal and chemical bodily adaptations.

Emotions have three components: subjective, behavioral, and physiological. The physiological correlates of stress are seen in the anxious patient, since anxiety and fear illicit the same bodily response. The GAS includes autonomic body changes that occur below the level of awareness or control (as flushing, perspiring, muscle tightening and tremors). These autonomic changes provide the nurse significant guides in inferences of the degree of a patient's "dis-stress".

Stress becomes maladaptive when there are too many life changes within a short time span, prohibiting the time required for accomodation and adjustment. Life change units (Holmes and Rahe) provide a means of assessing the total score of changes within a given time span and provide the nurse a useful assessment tool for primary prevention.

In written Chinese, the characters for crisis represent "opportunity" and "danger". While change is essential to life, planned change, within time constraints for adaptation, provides for growth; too many changes too quickly create dangerous system overload and crises. Anxiety evolves when a person experiences change from his habitual adaptive stance. As long as the emotional energy remains "free-floating" and unbound, the change is an opportunity for growth. Once attached to unconscious mechanisms that relieve the discomfort of stress, protecting the person's ego from the pain of anxiety, and rendering him "comfortable, but not well", change becomes crisis then unhealthy adaptation.

An innovative suggestion for the application of the GAS to nursing care plans uses seven objectives for nursing intervention and the GAS as a basis for a nursing approach. The five levels of adaptation point up the patient's strengths as well as needs:

First level: Reduction of primary stress by physiological and/or psychological adaptations. Rarely reaching conscious awareness, these are normal defense responses to stress, the healthy use of one's repertoire of defense mechanisms.

Second level: Adaptations that require a general awareness that something is amiss, i.e., signal anxiety. Person uses compensatory adaptations to control and limit stress.

Third level: Nonspecific generalized responses that are neither defensive nor compensatory occur as the person cannot limit, reduce, or control the stress. These are the signs and symptoms of health problems. Psychologically, anxiety conversions present such physical symptoms as headache, fatigue, and changes in physiology.

Fourth level: Third level adaptations create new stresses that require additional adaptation. Without outside intervention to halt the GAS, irreversible damage occurs (as continued elevated blood pressure causing permanent damage to the heart and blood vessels) with a state of panic, reality distortion and decreased comprehension.

Fifth level: Stresses are multiple, nursing intervention must reverse the GAS for survival. Acute phase of illness in psychological realm, usual defenses don't reduce anxiety, can adapt no longer and withdraws from reality (Saxton and Hyland, pp. 28-34).

Objectives of the nursing approach related to stress are:

1. Reduce or limit the extent and intensity of the present stress.
2. Prevent additional stress. Objectives related to the individual's level of adaptation are:
3. Support the individual's first level adaptations to assist in sustaining and maintaining defensive responses.
4. Limit and support the individual's second level adaptations to confine compensatory reactions.
5. Alter, limit and support the individual's third level adaptations to modify response symptoms.

6. Interrupt, alter, limit and support fourth level adaptation to intervene in stressors.
7. Supplement, interrupt, alter and limit the fifth level adaptation to complement or replace responses failing to control stress.

By controlling one's life change score, change can be pleasant and growth facilitating. Some of the steps for successfully accommodating to change are (O'Neill, 1974):

1. Exploration of the physical and psychological responses as one accommodates to change (as insomnia, overeating, anorexia), unifying the behavioral and physiological aspects with cognitive awareness.
2. Establish positive attitudes, working through blaming others, ruminating on past injustices to assuming responsibility for self.
3. "Center and focus" on own feelings, identity and life goals, finding the stable center of self by consciousness raising.
4. Share decision making with others who will help modify and validate accurate perceptions.
5. Organize a plan of action within time intervals.
6. Risk taking, careful exploration of alternates.
7. Gradual release of the problem by accommodation to newer, more acceptable attitudes and behaviors.

In the present technological society, changes occur so rapidly and frequently that preventative measures are necessary in order to avoid unmanageable stress.

REVIEW QUESTIONS

1. What are "dynamics" and of what use are they?
2. How do the levels of consciousness differ?
3. What are the functions of the Id, Ego, and Superego?
4. Identify the various defense mechanisms that you have used today.
5. What is the basic difference between suppression and repression?
6. In what order does Maslow feel that needs are met? Can you satisfy third level needs before second level needs?
7. How do conflict, stress, and frustration influence behavior?
8. Can you change behavior? How?

SUGGESTED REFERENCES

1. Bennis, W. G., et al.: The Planning of Change: Readings in the Applied Behavioral Sciences, Holt, Rinehart & Winston, New York, 1969

2. Benson, H.: Your innate asset for combating stress, Nursing Digest III:292-298, May-June, 1975

3. Bird, B.: Notes on transference: Universal phenomenon and hardest part of analysis, J Am Psychoanalytic Assoc XX:267-301, 1972

4. Cleland, V.: The effect of stress on performance, Nursing Research IV:292-298, Fall, 1975

5. Coombe, E.: Tuning in on stress signals, J Nursing Education IV:16-21, July, 1976

6. Davidhizar, R.H.: Stress patients: A new dimension in psychiatric nursing education, Perspectives in Psychi Care III:129-131, 1973

7. Defense Mechanisms, Programmed Text, Am J Nursing, Sept., 1972

8. Erickson, E.: Nursing--skilled work or a profession? International Nursing Review, Issue 208, IV:118-120, July-Aug., 1976

9. Freud, A.: The Ego and the Mechanisms of Defense, Hogarth Press, London, 1952

10. Harrison, V.: Linderman's crisis theory and Dabrowski's positive disintegration theory: A comparative analysis, Perspectives in Psychi Care VI:8, 1965

11. Holmes, T.H. and Rahe: Social readjustment rating scales, J Psychosom Research XI:213-218, 1967

12. James, M.: Development and transference factors, International J Psychoanalytic Psychother II:52-77, May, 1972

13. Jensen, D.J.: Crisis resolved: Impact through planned change, Nursing Clinics N Am IV:735-742, 1973

14. Johnson, R.: The blotting paper syndrome--a counter transference phenomenon, Perspectives in Psychi Care V:228, 1967

15. Koles, W.: Counter transference: A bilateral phenomenon in the learning model, Perspectives in Psychi Care VI:152, 1968

16. Lidz, T.: The Person, Basic Books, Inc., New York, 1970

17. Maslow, A.H.: Motivation and Personality, Harper & Bros., New York, 1954

18. Maslow, A.H.: Toward a Psychology of Being, Van Nostrand, Princeton, N. J., 1968

19. McGrath, Joseph (Ed.): Social and Psychological Factors in Stress, Holt, Rinehart & Winston, Inc., New York, 1970

20. O'Neill, N. and O'Neill, G.: Shifting Gears, Avon, New York, 1974

21. Pesznecker, B.: Life change: A challenge for nurse practitioners, Nurse Practitioner I:21-25, 1975

22. Reinkemeyer, A.M.: Nursing's need: A commitment to an ideology of change, Nursing Forum IV:340-355, 1970

23. Rogers, C. R. : On Becoming a Person, Houghton Mifflin Co. , Boston. 1961

24. Rodgers, J.A.: Theoretical considerations involved in the process of change, Nursing Forum XII:160-174, 1973

25. Saxton, D. F. and Hyland P. : Planning and Implementing Nursing Intervention, St. Louis, 1975

26. Seyle, H.: Stress Without Distress, McGraw Hill Book Co., Inc., New York, 1973

27. Seyle, H.: The Stress of Life, McGraw Hill Book Co., Inc., New York, 1956

28. Toffer, A.: Future Shock, Random House, New York, 1970

29. Veninga, R.: Defensive behavior: Causes, effects, and cures, Nursing Digest III:58-59, May-June, 1975

30. Wallis, G.G.: Stress as a predictor of schizophrenia, Br J Psychi CXX:375-384, 1972

31. Wheelis, A.: How people change, Commentary, May, 1969

CHAPTER 3

NURSING FUNCTIONS

In psychiatric nursing, patient care is centered in nurse-patient relationships. These relationships may be of different types:

1. Rooster: One is dominated and controlled by the other. The dominant one may not always be the nurse. A manipulative patient can control a nurse who wishes to be controlled.
2. Leech: Complete and total dependency upon the nurse. May also be reversed - nurse may be dependent to satisfy own needs with the patient.
3. Chimpanzee: Supportive relationship in which the weaker member can grow without fear or threat. A helping relationship.

THE HELPING RELATIONSHIP

A helping relationship involves more than just a supportive attitude on the part of the nurse. The patient's perceptions of the relationship are equally as important.

If the nurse sees herself as something the patient does not, there is not a helping relationship.

What is a helping relationship then? Some of Rogers' listed characteristics were:

1. Congruent: (The nurse is viewed as trustworthy, dependable and consistent).
2. Unambiguous: (The nurse is expressive and does not communicate contradictory messages).
3. Positive: (The nurse can experience positive feelings or attitudes toward the patient - love, warmth, caring, respect).
4. Strong: (The nurse needs to be strong enough as an individual to remain separate from the patient).
5. Secure: (The nurse needs to be secure enough to permit the patient to remain separate).
6. Empathic: (The nurse can enter into the patient's world and see it from his viewpoint).
7. Accepting: (The nurse can accept the patient as he is and can communicate the acceptance).
8. Sensitive: (The nurse is sensitive enough not to display behavior seen as threatening by the patient).
9. Nonjudgmental: (The nurse can refrain from evaluating or appearing to evaluate the patient).
10. Creative: (The nurse views the patient as a person in the process of "becoming" and not bound by his past).

The helping relationship is only one of the nursing functions of the modern psychiatric nurse. She must also be skilled in observation, communication and uses a deliberate rather than an intuitive nursing process.

THE NURSING PROCESS

Psychiatric nurses were the forerunners in applying a disciplined, intellectual approach to the nursing process. In recent years, process commonalities that cross all clinical nursing areas have been identified for a foundation of nursing practice. The problem-solving, decision-making sequential steps are:

1. Data collection
2. Nursing diagnosis
3. Plan for nursing action
4. Implementation of the plan
5. Evaluation of effectiveness

Recordings of the interpersonal nurse-patient process are a major tool for psychiatric nurses to analyze and implement the communication process. This process involves:

1. Analysis of the patient by collection of data of the patient's total needs through observation and assessment of the physical, psychological, social and environmental domains, pattern recognition and hypotheses formulation.
2. Selection of priorities for nursing care. From hypotheses, priorities are determined and ranked.
3. Selection of type of treatment and therapeutic strategies, established in collaboration with other health workers and with the client, encouraging the client to use his own resources for self-actualization.

The nursing process has four basic operations:

1. Observation of the patient, noting behavioral cues, facts and occurrences.
2. Inferences or interpretations drawn from these observations.
3. Interventions based on inferences, and
4. Evaluations of outcomes and reformulations of hypotheses.

The nursing diagnosis (a process of clinical inferences from observed changes in the patient's condition) leads to the identification of the possible causes of the symptomology. Nursing diagnosis has been identified as the "weakest link" in the nursing process (Aspinella, 1976). Since inferences in the areas of psychological states are more subtle and complex than in the physical realm (Peplau, 1959), the conscious, cognitive nursing process is the basis of effective psychiatric nursing care.

OBSERVATION

Observation is an active process utilizing all of the senses for the purpose of collecting data in order to make more accurate diagnoses. Observational data collected by any individual is the result of the individual's past experience, present situation, and expertise in observing. Effective observations are:

1. Nonjudgmental (honest and impersonal in both intent and prac-
    tice): the subject is not observed only at his worst nor with a
    preconceived bias. Behavior (window-breaking, cursing, fight-
    ing) is the same no matter who does it even though the meaning
    varies.
2. Goal-directed (done for an identified reason): the observations
    may be to assess the general appearance or behavior of the pa-
    tient or to focus upon the patient's eating habits, hand movements,
    etc. but are never just to while away the time or to satisfy idle
    curiosity.
3. Planned (done at specific times for specific periods and with spe-
    cific intervals between): observations are not done on a social
    "just passing by" basis. They are part of the therapeutic rela-
    tionship and are arranged for maximum effectiveness as is any
    other phase of nursing care.

Observations are made to facilitate recognition of behavior and plan
nursing care.

Observations are influenced by the observer. Just being there will
alter any given situation. No two people will ever observe a situation or an individual in exactly the same way. Observations are colored by the observer's personal biases and observers tend to notice
behaviors that are unexpected or unfamiliar. Observations focus on
those behaviors communicated nonverbally.

How observations are described is important. Not all observations
will be objective but they can be described clearly, concisely, and
specifically. Interpretations of the observed behaviors often differ.
Observations, once made, need to be recorded:

1. Use simple language, not psychiatric jargon.
2. Keep interpretation to a minimum.
3. Be clear and concise.
4. Be specific.
5. Be as objective as possible.
6. Record as soon as possible.

Recorded observations are communicated data.

COMMUNICATION

Communication is the process by which people exchange information,
share views, and express themselves in a reciprocal relationship.
In any reciprocal relationship:

1. The atmosphere created by the nurse will affect the interaction.
2. The nurse defines the needs and goals of the interaction.
3. The areas of conflict need to be resolved, if possible, or at least
    identified.
4. The needs and goals are continuously evaluated in terms of be-
    havior change.

Communication is of two kinds:

1. Verbal
2. Nonverbal

Verbal communication is dependent upon words, written or oral, to convey information and to respond.

NONVERBAL COMMUNICATION

Speechless messages are sent by vocal, facial, and gestural signals; they are received through the sense organs. Though all the senses are involved in nonverbal communication, visual perception has been given the most emphasis and is used interchangeably with the term observation. However, observation is the objective assessment of behavior; nonverbal communication includes the processes of sensing (detecting), identifying (differentiating), and cognitive interpretation. Verbal and nonverbal language do not use the same sense modalities, and whenever patients cannot use verbal language, nonverbal communication should be encouraged to keep communication lines open. "One picture is worth a thousand words" is true because:

1. Much of the nonverbal communication occurs outside the focus of attention and impinges subliminally and unconsciously on the eye of the beholder;
2. Language has not had descriptive terms to label, describe, and quantify the forms of nonverbal behaviors;
3. Nonverbal communication modes are combined or "patterned" for receptive inferences and the combinations and different intensities of nonverbal patterns lack identification and descriptive language.

Much of nursing arts and science relies on non-verbal indices for patient problem identification. In most life-threatening patient conditions, the nurse relies on disease signs and symptoms and nonverbal cues for clinical inferences. Since limitations in language limit both the use of spoken and written words to describe nonverbal cues, nursing students are given essential clinical practice opportunities to observe clinical "role models" and apply theoretical concepts as well as learn by example, the "practice wisdom" of patient care. In the apprentice-type programs, student nurses nonverbally absorb the role model's use of the indescribable, yet essential nonverbal patient messages contributing to clinical inferences. In collegiate programs, "participant observation" roles are used involving the student observer silently in the interaction context. This detached presence puts the learner in touch with the nonverbal transaction by involving her sense modalities in experiential learning.

In psychiatric nursing, nonverbal communication is of special importance. Many emotional states are conveyed nonverbally, and troubling emotions usually occur below the patient's conscious, cognitive level. Through denial, repression and other defenses, patients are often not "in touch" with their emotions. Frequently, the task of the psychiatric nurse is to facilitate congruence between what is verbally and nonverbally communicated.

During the last few years, behavioral scientists have begun to evolve a "language" for nonverbal communication and these terms and labels are beginning to appear in the psychiatric nursing literature. Some of the terminology, definitions, and implications of these concepts for nursing are as follows:

1. Organismic: appearances, including physical trait groups as sex, race, age, and personal attractiveness. What is conveyed by organismic attributes is often "so loud" it drowns out the simultaneous verbal message. Human rights efforts for women, minorities, and the aged protest discrimination on organismic grounds. Rinkleman's research found psychiatric nurses are markedly influenced by organismic factors in patient perception, and these perceptions influence the quality of nursing care.

2. Adornment: conscious efforts made by the person to alter or enhance the physical image through cosmetics, jewelry, and wearing apparel. Self-presentation conveys mood by selection of style and color, revealing the person's "aspired image". Adornments have a status signalling function (as uniforms, stethoscopes, and tennis shoes) especially for men (blue-collar workers). Women's attire has traditionally been seductive, subject to cyclic exposure of various body parts and called "fashion". Adornment conveys appropriateness, outmodedness, conservativeness, outlandishness, and "individuality". Present day role blurring of masculine-feminine adornment is disturbing to the older generation who have traditionally relied on adornment for nonverbal communication of sex and role status.

3. Oculesics: refers to glances and eye movements conveying nonverbal information. Everyday body language and tradition attribute great power and mystery to the eyes -- they are the "portholes to the soul", one is given the "evil eye" or asked to "look directly in another's eye" so deception can be detected. The "mind's eye" is linked to verbal recall and the commonly used phrase, "I see" means "I understand". The "third" eye refers to "in-sight" gained by adhering to certain eastern religious practices and beliefs.

People use eye-contact to show they are paying attention and eye contact is a criterion frequently used as a sign of mental health. High status people usually get more visual attention than they give.

While most body expressions are learned and culture-bound, pupillometric changes, the dilating of the pupil when pleased ("wide-eyed") and constricting of the pupil when disturbed ("probing", "narrow", or "angry" eyes) is an unconscious, autonomic emotional reponse and is one of the most relied upon nonverbal indices nurses used to predict potential for emotional "explosion" and acting out (Clunn, 1975).

4. Facial Expressions: associated with emotion and used synonomously with eye expressions. However, except for the pupils, the eyes do not structurally change during emotion; the facial skin areas around the eyes do change. While facial expressions are the most commonly relied upon indices of nonverbal communication, research shows they are also the most deceptive and culturally different. Physiogromic structures vary and one's face is a "recognized" individual

characteristic. Individual facial repertoires also vary; not everyone can "raise an eyebrow" or "pull a poker face". There is common distrust of facial control; people say they "won't show their face" for fear the emotions they wish to hide will be unwittingly conveyed.

Blushing or "turning chalk white" happens only to the face and body surfaces exposed to the observing eye. Like pupillometric changes, blushing occurs below the blusher's level of awareness and is often laughingly called attention to by the observer. While blushing is usually accepted jovially as a "body give-away", other discrepancies between verbal and nonverbal messages evoke anger in the receiver, insulted to have the sender try to "pull the wool over his eyes". These ego defending angry reactions are common in psychiatric settings where the conflicting messages may be interpreted as the sender seeing the receiver as insensitive or dull. Whenever there are discrepancies between verbal and nonverbal messages, credence is given to the nonverbal; everyday wisdom knows "actions speak louder than words".

Research studies of facial expressions have been unable to identify cross-cultural, universal affect expressions, except for the upward lifting of the corners of the mouth, a universal expression of pleasure currently enjoying great popularity in the "Happy Face" symbol. However, recent cross cultural studies (Eckman, et al.) of facial expressions of happiness, sadness, surprise, anger, and disgust report these have more universal facial similarity than previously believed.

5. Chronemics: nonverbal messages conveyed by the use of time are illustrated by who waits for whom and how long, (as people waiting hours in physicians' offices). Those who "fill-up" the most time talking in conversations believe themselves to be the most important in the interaction. Silences used can indicate boredom or be attention getting. Time pauses can mark the conclusion of a topic or the punctuation of an important message as: Listen for the following, important announcement.

Timing is often attributed to natural impingements beyond the control of the person. "Poor timing" is a common rationalization for out of sequence errors. Timing in the psychotherapeutic process refers to introjections and confrontations judiciously guided by nonverbal indices of the patients' "readiness" to positively assimilate and accommodate to the information.

6. Vocalics and Paralinguistics: describe how things are said, the context of communication in contrast to the content of the verbalization. Voice conveys personality and the state of an interaction: repetitions, slurs, stuttering and hesitations are para-language indications of affect. Researchers have studied paralanguage by having subjects read "content free" material (as the alphabet) to isolate the affective transmission through verbalization rather than word content (Davitz). The discrepancies between content and context also underlie the "double bind" of communication theory. Paralanguage is of special interest to researchers of how young children learn to speak, and research findings indicate the first approximations are molded and structured by significant others and that paralanguage is an essential precursor to the development of verbal language.

Psychiatric patients with limited verbal communication are often also inept in the nonverbal supportive paralinguistic components of verbal transactions. They may need guidance in developing congruent expressive nonverbal speech as well as awareness of the signals and rules for taking turns in speaking conversations.

7. Objectics: are objects and personal belongings that people surround themselves with and are experienced as extensions or expressions of the self-image. Ash trays, coffee cups, brief cases, motorcycles and/or sports cars convey things about the person's selection, choice, and emotional investment in objects.

During home visits, the nurse has opportunities to observe furnishings and home decor which nonverbally communicate what and how objects are valued. The collecting of specific classes of objects reveal personal interests and each person and family have "relics" from their past that provide historical insights to the observer.

8. Kinesic Communication: is the communication of feeling by postures, positions and movements that occur between body movements and repositioning. Of the many detailed descriptions of the meaning of kinesics, a general summary is that extended, loose limbs imply relaxed, open states and contracted, restricted, "close to the body" limb positioning imply fear, anxiety and "protection" of self. Slumped posture with sagging muscles conveys the message of being "burdened with the weight of the world" on one's back or the need to "get something off the chest" that pulls the frame forward and downward; the opposite "stiff-backed", upright posture conveys strict propriety. Common parlance currently uses the term "posture" in nonverbal communication terms, i.e., the position taken toward an abstract concept.

The filtration of nonverbal communication language into everyday speech is reflected by the numerous lay books flooding the market, as Body Language and How to Read a Person Like a Book. The popularity of these books stems from the general awareness that "there's more to life than what meets the eye", and a highly mobile society's need to find quicker, more reliable tactics in forming friendships. Traditionally, low mobility provided leisure time for familiarity and trust between people to evolve slowly. Caution should be exercised in superficially attributing emotional meaning to a specific stance (as arms folded across the chest interpreted as uninvolved indifference). Understanding a person's nonverbal communication requires knowledge of cultural differences, idiosyncracies, past and present situations and inclusion of other nonverbal, supportive cues and pattern response replication.

9. Interactional Synchrony: refers to coordinated and/or "out of tune" kinesic movements exchanged between persons in verbal and nonverbal interactions. These synchronous movements may be partially directed by speech; however, the coordinating movements of social interaction can be without eye contact or the use of words. Both speaker and listener perform a "conversation dance", and research analysis of slow motion films illustrates the elaborate feedback in conversation concert (Condon and Ogston). The listener, as a shadow of speech, moves in harmony, indicating his synchrony

with the speaker, or disharmony and being "out of step". That people "march to different tunes" has heretofore been merely a beautiful poetic description; recent research makes this disharmony a visible reality.

Film studies of psychotherapy sessions show harmonious non-verbal communication interaction patterns during fruitful session. Body movements often precede verbal content, relating directly or symbolically to the nonverbal actions. For example, a client's arm twitched prior to his statement that he "felt like hitting someone" (Ekman).

Infant research findings show kinesic synchrony develops from the mother-child interaction and that normal infants have highly developed nonverbal communication repertoires. These are essential foundations for speech development. Psychiatric patients frequently have had faulty parent relationships during infancy and this disruption may explain, in part, the "bizarre" unsynchronized behavior patterns which evolved "autistically", outside a sustained positive reinforcement pattern of parental validation.

Since kinesic synchrony underlies compatible productive interactions, the nurses' approach to patients should provide for "introduction time", preliminary opportunities for getting "in tune" with the patient. It has been suggested empathic synchrony can be more easily established by the practitioners' conscious mirroring of the patient's kinesic gestures. Getting "in tune" prior to reducing spatial proximity and to nursing intervention is especially important with small children, nonverbal, and psychiatric patients.

10. Proxemic Communication: uses space and structure in the silent language, while "territoriality" is the drive to maintain and defend the exclusive right to a piece of property. Everyone has interior space plans that determine their individual spatial tolerance. Space is related to feelings of freedom and vary according to situations. The limited "life space" of many hospitals add to patients' feelings of depersonalization and skillful management of the milieu requires a high degree of awareness of interpersonal movements and distancing as they affect emotional stability. The claustrophobic and the potentially explosive patient with a body buffer zone five times that of people at peace (Kinzel), manifests behaviors preventable by the nurse's "anticipatory" proxemic intervention. Kinesic synchronizations convey to the receiver the welcome -- or refusal -- to enter the body buffer zone and the proxemic mode of the person approached.

Four zones of spacial interaction are: close, intimate distance, personal and social. Nursing approaches should be based on assessment of the patient's mode of spacial interaction. Milieu management includes monitoring of patient's pain, anxiety and stress, and traffic flow. Many acting out behaviors are triggered by spacial confinement. Crowding in small areas triggers threats of depersonalization when weak ego boundaries are a problem.

11. Hapatic, Nonverbal Communication Through Touch: is probably the most basic form of human interaction and an important corner-

stone to the nursing practice of "laying on of hands". Sullivanian Theory stresses the psychological significance of touch in transmitting emotional tones that affect the development of trust. The self-concept has its roots in parental handling fostering feelings of acceptance and recognition. The "good me"; in the anxious, abrasive painful touching leading to the "bad me"; and the extreme, dissociated tactile messages forming the uncanny "not me" personifications.

Instinctual bonds of attachment, formed through sight, sound, and touch are described by Bowlby as the essential framework for later separation and ego individuation. By attachment bonds, the mother safely supports the child in learning the basics of life - feelings, cognition, and goal-directed behaviors. Studies of infant monkeys and humans suggest early tactile experience determines later intellectual, social and emotional development.

The mother's initial bonding weakens as the child matures, yet she needs to be available as a supportive, tactile "safety" reinforcer. Long after ego boundaries have been defined, the child "regressively" runs to mother to have her "kiss" a cut or bruise, or hold him close to take away the pain of "hurt feelings" or anxiety. The notion that a nurturing person can absorb or share pain through body contact is demonstrated by adults during times of emotional intensity and grief. Embraces, tightly squeezing another's hand, reassuring "pats on the back", and strokes as well as pushing and striking others are non-verbal communication of feelings by body contact.

The delicate, judicious and appropriate use of Touch is the art of nursing. Sometimes patients regress to the level of the sick, frightened children when they experience pain and anxiety. For some, the fear of losing their independent and separate identity is terrifying, stirring sentiments of past ties and dependencies. They struggle to maintain their ego boundaries. At such times, the nurse's use of touch is counterproductive to the patients' self-actualizing defenses against regressive tendencies, his need to maintain his ego differentiation. Nurses' indiscriminately touching patients without a prior positive trust relationship can be abrasive to patients, transmitting sensations stimulating the "bad me" or "not me" mode. Thus, the nurse can unwittingly "touch-off" more pain or an emotional explosion. Nursing approaches should sustain patients in their efforts to maintain ego differentiation or communicate support. The "laying on of hands" is a delicate nursing prerogative, exquisite in its healing or hurting potential.

The "use of self" in nursing is often more nonverbal than verbal. Feelings may be communicated by gestures, by expressions, by movement, and by words.

The most important communication between nurse and patient may well be "the approach". Approach refers to the way in which the nurse becomes closer to the patient for the express purpose of providing nursing care and planning further treatment goals.

If the nurse acts upon observations and interpretations of the meanings of observed behaviors or feelings, the interpretations need to be correct from the patient's viewpoint. Only the patient knows the meaning of his behavior and his feelings to him, and it is the patient's perceptions that matter.

Before acting upon any interpretations, the nurse seeks validation from the patient. If the patient appears angry, the nurse can check with the patient to see whether her interpretation is right or wrong. By seeking such validation, the nurse obtains more accurate data for effective planning, and the patient sees that someone is trying to understand his feelings from his point of view. This feeling of being understood and accepted is the essence of a helping or therapeutic relationship. The nurse may use verbal or physical approaches or a combination of both.

When planning the approach the nurse needs to consider:

1. The nurse (Why approach this patient? For what purpose?)
2. The patient (How will he perceive the situation? What is the best approach?)
3. The purpose (What is the immediate purpose? What are the long-range goals?)

One of the most important components of effective communication is the ability to listen. Listening is an active act, not a passive one. Listening is focused on the content and the feeling being communicated, not on the comment to be made at the first pause. An effective listener "hears" the words that are not uttered, "hears" the clenching of hands that are not seen, "hears" the silence. An effective listener hears his own words, spoken and unspoken, as well as those of others. The effective listener becomes a participant observer taking an active role in the interaction.

Communication is always a two-way process. Both the patient and the nurse need to listen and to talk, to write and to read.

THE SELF-CONCEPT AND INTERPERSONAL PERCEPTIONS

The meaning of the patient's behavior to the patient is the only relevant basis on which the nurse can formulate a plan of care (Peplau). The self-concept is the perception a person holds of himself, an internal frame of reference which describes who he is, what he does, and how he feels about himself. Additional definitions describe the self-concept as:

The evaluation of one's accomplishments, abilities, and worth.

A permanent, consistent position in the phemenological field identified as self viewed by interactions with others, the external frame of reference.

A conscious and unconscious mirror-image of self that is communicated verbally and nonverbally.

An internal frame of reference of self affecting how others are perceived and interacted with.

An organizer and integrater of experience and behavior.

While self-concept and ego are used interchangeably, most theorists say the two are not synonomous; the self-concept is an object, the ego a process of self identity and self evaluation.

The self-concept responds selectively to experience to maintain its "integrity". Research (Fitts) comparing the self-concepts of "normals" and persons with psychopathology show significant differences, and the self-concept is considered a valid index of mental illness.

Knowledge of a person's self-concept is basic to understanding his behavior since many aspects of behavior correlate with the self-concept. How one sees himself influences how one perceives and reacts to the world around him. If the nurse knows the patient's self-concept, much can be predicted about his behavior; self-perceptions clarify how much the patient will participate in self-actualization: the more optimal the self-concept, the more effectively the person will function; the more dissonance between identity and isolated self, the more disintegration occurs. The weaker the self-image, the more likely the distortions in how he perceives and interacts with the world around him.

To help the patient, the nurse must know how he sees himself and how he views his situation. The nurse needs to clarify how he sees his situation and problem; and the patient's way of viewing the problem is governed by his concept of self and the skills he has available to tackle the tasks of reintegration.

The following have been suggested as useful in assessing the self-concept:

1. Have patient describe his perception of his physical appearance.
2. Have patient describe his perception of his self-worth.
3. Have patient describe his perception of his body image.
4. Have patient describe his perception of his role in family and community.
5. Have patient describe his perception of his role as patient.

These perceptions should be compared with others' perceptions of the patient - staff, family, friends, other patients - and descriptions identified (Simmons).

The higher the nurse's interpersonal accuracy of the patient's self-concept, the more successful the intervention. This accuracy directs the nurse's empathy and language to be attuned to the client's feelings.

Outcomes of therapeutic interventions are generally stated in "improvements" or reorganization of the self-concept through therapy. Carl Rogers notes the following effects of therapy on the self-concept:

1. The perception of self is the aspect of personality most radically changed in therapy.
2. The changes appear to be more in the meanings given things (stimuli) than the things themselves.
3. The self the person wants to be (idealized self) is reorganized to a lesser degree in therapy.
4. The idealized self-image and the real self are more congruent.
5. There is more confidence in the reorganized self.

Other theorists noting the reorganization of perception of self as a result of therapy add:

1. Increased self-esteem
2. Less dependent on the evaluation of self and more dependent on the experience of self
3. Increased awareness of self with less distortion of sensory data.
4. Increased ability to be objective in evaluating one's ability, characteristics, and self in relation to others.
5. Increased ability to perceive self as evaluator of experiences.

Before the nurse intervenes, validation with the patient of assumed behavioral meanings is necessary. If nurse and patient interpret differently, progress is minimal, and probably accidental. The process of identifying, validating, and changing inappropriate non-productive behavior is purposeful and rewarding for both nurse and patient, enhancing their development as members of humanity.

INTERVENTION

Nursing intervention differs from problem solving; intervention deals with the patient in his entire situation, while problem solving deals with a specific issue. Two prerequisites for intervention are:

1. Knowledge of behavioral and biological sciences.
2. Skill in communication, reasoning and hypothesis formulation.

A developmental, conceptual framework for the steps in intervention that provides a baseline for nursing actions (Gorman and McClean, 1966), is as follows:

1. Assessment: drawn from acquired knowledge of the patient's situation; the general meaning, complexity and patient's identifiable needs. Then,
2. Judgment: made on the basis of the assessment as to the need for intervention. If intervention is needed,
3. Goal Setting: tentative, immediate, or long-term, preventative, supportive, or therapeutic in nature.
4. Selection: an effective, appropriate intervening behavior and approach is determined.

5. Choice of Agent: most suitable person for intervention is selected (if referral, nurse takes secondary role) if nurse decides she's suitable, then,
6. Action: preventative, supportive, or therapeutic intervention in patient's situation is taken.
7. Evaluation: of patient's response to action, followed by
8. Reassessment: of patient's situation.
9. Set Tentative Goals: and a nursing care plan. If rejected, then reassessment of the patient's situation and new hypothesis are formulated.
10. Conclusion: nurse follows process to its conclusion; and a) patient moves to independence, situation resolved; or b) referral to suitable agent is made.

REVIEW QUESTIONS

1. What is a helping relationship?
2. What are the three types of patient-nurse relationships?
3. What does "congruent" mean?
4. What is the purpose of observing patients?
5. Many things affect individual observation. What are some of them?
6. What are the attributes of an effective observation?
7. Of what use are exterior signs? What are some of the exterior signs?
8. How can time and space be observed?
9. How are expressive behaviors evaluated?
10. How are observations communicated?
11. What are some of the components of a successful communication?
12. What is an approach"?

SUGGESTED REFERENCES

1. Aden, G.: There are no mute patients, In Some Clinical Approaches to Psychiatric Nursing, Bued & Marshall, Eds., The Macmillan Co., New York, 1963

2. Aspinella, M.J.: Nursing diagnosis - The weakest link, Nursing Outlook XXIV:433-437, July, 1976

3. Birdwhistell, R.L.: Kinesics and Context, University of Pennsylvania Press, Philadelphia, 1970

4. Bowlby, J.: Attachment and loss, Vol. I: Attachment, International Psychoanalytic, Hogart Press Library, London, 1969

5. Brown, R.A.: A First Language: The Early Stages, Harvard University Press, Cambridge, 1973

6. Byers, V.: Nursing Observations, W.C. Brown Co., Iowa, 1968 V

7. Clunn, P.A.: Nurse's Assessment of a Person's Potential for Violence, Teachers College, Columbia University, Doctoral Dissertation, 1975

8. Condon, U.S.: Movement of awake-active neonates demonstrated to synchronize with adult speech, Paper presented at the biennial meeting of the Society for Research in Child Development, Philadelphia, Pennsylvania, March, 1973

9. Cooley, C.H.: Looking glass self, Symbolic Interaction, Nanis, J.G. and Melzer, B.M., Eds., Allyn & Bacon, Boston, 1967

10. Davitz, J.R. and Davitz, L.J.: The communication of feelings by content free speech, J Communication IX:6-13, 1959

11. Davitz, J.R.: A dictionary and grammar of emotion, Arnold, M., Ed., Feelings and Emotions, Academic Press, New York, 1970

12. Dominian, J.: The psychological significance of touch, Nursing Times, pp. 29-32, July 22, 1971

13. Ducan, S.: Some signals and rules for taking speaking turns in conversation, J Personality Social Psychol XXIII:283-292, 1972

14. Ekman, P. and Friesen, W.V.: Nonverbal leakage and clues to deception, Psychiatry CXXXII:88-109, 1969

15. Ekman, P. and Friesen, W.V.: Nonverbal behavior in psychotherapy research, In Research in Psychotherapy, Vol. III, Shlien, J.M., Ed., American Psychological Association, Washington, D.C., pp. 179-216, 1968

16. Fast, J.: Body Language, Pocket Books, New York, 1971

17. Fisher, S.: Body Consciousness, Jason Aronson, New York, 1973

18. Fitts, W.H.: The Self-Concept and Behavior: Overview and Supplement, Research Monograph No. 7, The Dade Wallace Center, Nashville, Tenn., June, 1972

19. Fitts, W.H.: The Self-Concept and Performance, Research Monograph No. 5, The Dade Wallace Center, Nashville, Tenn., April, 1972

20. Fitts, W.H.: The Self-Concept and Psychopathology, Research Monograph No. 4, The Dade Wallace Center, Nashville, Tenn., March, 1972

21. Gebbie, K. and Lavin, M. A.: Classifying nursing diagnosis, Am J Nursing, Feb., 1974

22. Goffman, E.: Presentation of Self in Everyday Life, Anchor Books, New York, 1966

23. Gorman, M. L. and McClean, L.: Towards a definition of intervention, Interpersonal Relationships, Maloney, E., Ed., William Brown Co., Dubuque, Iowa, pp. 54-72, 1966

24. Guller, I.B.: Stability of the self-concept in schizophrenia, J Abnormal Psychol LXXXI:275-279, April, 1966

25. Hays, J. and Larson, K.: Interaction with Patients, The Macmillan Co., New York, 1963

26. Kinzel, A.F.: Body-buffer zone in violent prisoners, Am J Psychi CXXVII:99-104, 1970

27. Koehne-Kaplan, N.S. and Tilden, V.P.: The process of clinical judgment in nursing practice: The component of personality, Nursing Research XXV:268-272, July-Aug., 1976

28. Kratz, C.R.: Participant observation in dyadic and triadic situations, International J Nursing Studies XII:169-174, 1976

29. Maloney, E., Ed.: How to play the territorial game, Perspectives in Psychi Care X:31, 1972

30. Montagu, A.: Touching, Columbia University Press, New York, 1971

31. Newman, M.: Movement tempo and the experience of time, Nursing Research CXXV:273-279, July-Aug., 1976

32. Nierenberg, G.J. and Calero, H.H.: How to Read a Person Like a Book, Hawthorne, New York, 1971

33. Orlando, I.J.: The Dynamic Nurse-Patient Relationship, G.P. Putnam & Sons, New York, 1961

34. Peplau, H.E.: Interpersonal Relations in Nursing, G.P. Putnam & Sons, New York, 1952

35. Phillips, R.: Language in disguise, nonverbal communication with patients, Perspectives Psychi Care IV:18, 1966

36. Pluckham, M.: Space: The silent language, Nursing Forum VII: 386-397, 1968

37. Reik, T.: Listening with the Third Ear, Grove Press, New York, 1956

38. Rinkelman, B.: Characteristics of Nurses and of Psychiatric Patients to whom they React Positively and Negatively, Doctoral Dissertation, Teacher's College, Columbia University, 1973

39. Rogers, C.R.: The necessary and sufficient conditions of therapeutic personality change, J Consulting Clinical Psychol XXI: 95-103, 1957

40. Rogers, C.R., Ed.: The Therapeutic Relationship and Its Impact, University of Wisconsin Press, Madison, Wisc., 1967

41. Scheflen, A.: How Behavior Means, Jason Aronson, New York, 1974

42. Simmons, J.A.: Self-image, Chapter 6, The Nurse-Patient Relationship in Psychiatric Nursing, W.B. Saunders, Philadelphia, pp. 95-106, 1969

43. Skipper, J.K. and Leonard, R.C.: Social Interaction and Patient Care, J.B. Lippincott Co., Philadelphia, 1965

44. Smith, D.W.: Change: How shall we respond to it? Nursing Forum IX:391-399, 1970

45. Suarez, R.: The silent patient in group therapy, J Psychi Nursing Mental Health Services, pp. 12-19, July-Aug., 1970

46. Tagiuri, R. and Petrullio, L.: Person Perception and Interpersonal Behavior, Stanford University Press, Stanford, Calif., 1958

47. Tragu, G.P.: A first approximation, Studies in Linguistics XIII: 1-12, 1958

48. Travelbee, J.: Interpersonal Aspects of Nursing, Davis, F.A., 2nd Ed., Philadelphia, 1971

49. Ward, J.T.: The sounds of silence, Perspectives Psychi Care XII:13-19, 1974

50. Weitz, S., Ed.: Nonverbal Communication, Oxford University Press, New York, 1974

CHAPTER 4

DEVELOPMENTAL THEORIES

Some knowledge of basic human development is necessary in order to understand people who are functioning with inappropriate or ineffective behavioral responses.

Developmental theories that stress stages of development help to point out that a behavior is appropriate or inappropriate as related to the individual's stage. Behavior has no meaning in isolation; "thumb sucking" cannot be interpreted except in relationship to development. A given behavior has different meaning during infancy than during childhood. No behavior has only one meaning (see Appendix B).

Some theorists stress the internal determination of development and the importance of successfully completing one stage before attempting the next. Other theorists stress external influences on development and the importance of interpersonal relationships in modifying behaviors from an unsuccessfully completed stage during a later stage.

Theorists may utilize the concepts of Id, Ego, and Superego as basic components of development. Energy, tension, conflict, anxiety - all related to behavior - have their own place in development theory. Although there are many theories of personality development based upon these concepts, Piaget is the only developmental theorist to focus upon cognitive development.

Four of the leading proponents of development by stages are:

1. S. Freud
2. H. S. Sullivan
3. E. Erikson
4. J. Piaget

S. FREUD

Freud was perhaps the first theorist to stress development by stages and the influence of early childhood experiences upon adult behavior. He felt that the first five years were the most important, that after the age of five the basic character was already formed.

Of Freud's five stages, three are presumably completed before the age of five. No one stage is ever completely replaced by another and residues of all stages are found in adults. Freud's dynamics of personality:

1. Structural hypothesis: The distribution and use of psychic energy by the functional structures of the mind - Ego, Id, Superego.
2. Psychic energy: The force behind mental activity arising originally from the Id and later diverted to the Ego or Superego.

3. Cathexis: The capacity of the psychic energy to be attracted or repelled by environmental objects which are then invested with special significance or feeling for the individual.
4. Object cathexis: The investment of psychic energy in an object (or in its symbolic representation) outside the individual which will gratify the Id (security blanket, parents, alcohol).
5. Anticathexis: The investment of psychic energy by the Ego to control Id impulses (dieting, thinking logically, going "on the wagon").
6. Tension: The driving forces of the Id (cathexis) are countered by the restraining forces of the Ego (anticathexis) resulting in personality conflicts.
7. Ego-cathexis: The psychic energy is displaced to objects only remotely associated with need (aggressive drives may be satisfied by hunting or by collecting guns or other weapons).
8. Ego defense mechanisms: The psychic energy is used to change the source (from Id to Ego by identification to Superego by introjection) or the object (by displacement).
9. Anxiety: The Ego is threatened by excessive stimulation which it can't control (temptation, guilt, shame).
10. Developmental stages: The psychic energy focuses in cathexis - anticathexis conflicts around the different erotogenic zones of the body.

The stages of development are five:

1. Oral stage: The mouth is the dynamic focus of energy during the first 18 months of life. At first, emphasis is passive:
   a. Receives food
   b. Does not actively meet needs
   c. Dependent on mother
   d. Sucking
   Later emphasis is active:
   a. Biting
   b. Talking
   c. Kissing
   These behaviors carry over into adult life and are recognized in later character traits, for example:
   a. The gullible individual who will "swallow" anything.
   b. The sarcastic individual with the "biting" wit.
2. Anal stage: Cathexis and anticathexis conflict focused on eliminative functions during the second 18 months. Toilet training during this time may greatly influence later traits.
   a. Strict training: child may hold back, become constipated, negative, stubborn, and stingy. Or he may aggressively expel feces anywhere at any time, become messy, destructive, cruel.
   b. Permissive training: child may consider bowel movements as important and desirable and become more outgoing, generous, productive, actively trying to please others.
   Behaviors from this stage are also recognizable in adult life:
   a. The miser, the compulsively clean individual, the common ordinary stamp collector.
   b. The aggressive he-man, the over-aged "hippie", the sadist.
   c. The creative artist, the sculptor, the philanthropist.

3. Phallic stage: Energy focus shifts to the genitals for the next two or three years. The superego develops and external values are internalized, especially the mother's values. As sexual activity becomes noticeable the child may be rewarded or punished.
   a. Punishment makes child feel guilty, dirty, shameful. Behavior not necessarily stopped but becomes more covert.
   b. Reward gives child the impression that sex is more important than other activities, or that sex can be sublimated in creative activities.
   c. Combination of reward and "punishment" may put sex in its proper perspective depending upon child's perception.

   These behaviors are also observable in adults:
   a. Pornography, censor, voyeur, deviant.
   b. Exhibitionist, Don Juan, writer, horticulturist.
   c. Middle-class American with usual acceptable hang-ups: nudity and sex occur in private but aren't discussed in public; homosexuality is destructive to the family unit; marriage should result in children.

   Two of the most important events in development occur during this stage. Freud felt his description of the Oedipal and castration complexes were his most important contributions to developmental theory.
   a. Oedipal complex: Cathexis (parent of the opposite sex), anticathexis (parent of the same sex) conflict. The little boy wishes to destroy his father and marry his mother. The little girl wishes to displace her mother and possess her father. The massive denial by the child at the oedipal stage leads to the full development of the repression mechanism, the cornerstone of all mental mechanisms.
   b. Castration complex: Boy fears father will castrate him for desiring mother. Girl is hostile towards mother because she feels castrated, develops cathexis for father's penis. (Penis envy is considered the female counterpart of castration anxiety).

   The Oedipal complex may be resolved or not resolved. Castration anxiety tends to help repress a boy's Oedipal conflict. A girl's conflict persists in modified form and is not totally repressed.

   Resolution of the Oedipal conflict is necessary for mature behavior. Theoretically the individual emerges from the conflict with a strong identification with the parent of the same sex. However, Freud assumed inherent bisexuality in everyone.

   Oedipal and castration conflicts left unresolved may be observable in adult life:
   a. Individuals who have problems with authority figures.
   b. Sexual deviants (i.e., homosexuality, incest).
   c. The weight-lifter and the chess player.
   d. Freud - who had a possessive dominating mother.

4. Latency stage: The prepubertal years are quiet years. The child is busy with school, friends, the world and his own interests. The earlier stages were egocentric, the child was interested in himself, his body, his parents, his pleasure. Now the child is more socialized, interested in external events.

   Energy is directed outward, the child strives to belong, to be one of the group, "homosexual".

Some of the behaviors of latency carry over into adult life:
a. Fraternity members
b. Conformists
c. Male chauvinist and women's lib
d. Male athletes and women volunteers
e. Gangs

5. Genital stage: Energy now focused on love-object of opposite sex. Period of identity crisis. Unable to define himself in relationship to others. This is the adolescent who is becoming more altruistic, more realistic, more concerned about the world but is egocentric and views the world through biased eyes.
Striving for independence, he may become aggressive or withdrawn, gregarious or a "loner".
During adolescence, learnings from the previous stages are integrated and fused into a realistic, adult, socialized behavior. Adolescent behaviors are observable in adults who have not resolved the conflicts of the early adolescent years, and also in those who retain the best of adolescent behaviors:
a. The rebel and the idealist.
b. The egotist and the reformer.
c. The hermit and the dreamer.
d. The inconsiderate and the empathic.

H. S. SULLIVAN

Sullivan used the concept of the conscious and unconscious mind, as did Freud. He stressed that individuals learned to behave in certain ways as a result if interpersonal relations.

Behavior patterns are called dynamisms and serve to satisfy the individual's basic needs. One dynamism, however, arises from anxiety and is called the self-system.

The self-system is formed from security measures adopted to protect the individual from anxiety and is, supposedly, the product of the more irrational aspects of the environmental culture. The self-system interferes with constructive changes in the personality by preventing objective assessment of behavior by the individual involved. The self-system, continually reinforced throughout life, becomes adept at protecting the personality from criticism by its real self. The self-system colors all experience.

Experience is of three cognitive modes:

1. Prototaxic: raw data from the senses, without meaning or relatedness (infant's first impressions of, and reactions to, his environment).
2. Parataxic: seeing causal relationships between events that are not logically related (whenever a riot occurs the police and/or students and/or hard hats, etc. are there, so obviously the police and/or students and/or hard hats, etc. cause riots). This thinking is basic to prejudice and discrimination.
3. Syntaxic: logical communication with symbols or language having the same meaning to all involved in the communication (accepted

as the logical mode of communication between "mature" individuals but is probably less common than parataxic).

As the child's self-system and experience develop he personifies first himself and then others with good-bad natures. The most recently met "others" become personifications of earlier similar personalities and are prejudged as good or bad depending upon previous experiences. Personifications help protect the self from anxiety by providing built-in bases for avoiding or controlling the bad or harmful others.

Personification of others, the self-system and the cognitive modes all affect (and are affected by) the interpersonal relationships that contribute to the development of personality. Throughout the life span those people who are most important to the individual, his "significant others", may be his family, his peers, his friends or his neighbors. They will help or hinder his total development. The stages of development are six:

1. Infancy: The mouth is zone of interpersonal activity. Develops concepts of the nipple:
   a. Good nipple (satisfaction in nursing).
   b. Unsatisfactory nipple (good nipple when not hungry).
   c. Wrong nipple (no milk).
   d. Bad nipple (avoidance of anxious mother).
   Other features of this stage:
   a. Change from prototaxic to parataxic modes.
   b. Beginning of self-system.
   c. Need satisfaction by self (thumb-sucking).
2. Childhood: The transition to childhood is made possible by acquisition of language. Some of the aspects of this stage:
   a. Self-system begins developing concept of gender.
   b. Use of syntaxic mode.
   c. Development of more coherent self-system.
   d. First feelings about others as enemies.
   e. Interpersonal relations colored by distrust of others, cultural view of sex role, and extent of language capabilities.
3. Juvenile era: Extending through most of grammar school. Some aspects:
   a. Internal control of behavior.
   b. Experience with authority figures outside the family.
   c. Group feeling, socialization.
   d. Distinguishing fantasy from reality.
   e. New methods of sublimation.
4. Preadolescence: A brief period centering around "best friend" or chum relationship. Other aspects:
   a. Interpersonal relationships move from older individuals to peers.
   b. Beginning of genuine interpersonal human relationships.
   c. Without best friend child becomes lonely and withdrawn or overaggressive.
5. Early adolescence: The energies are focused on developing heterosexual relationships:
   a. Mouth, hands, and genitals are zones of activity.
   b. Beginnings of feeling of lust.

   c. Erotic feelings directed toward the opposite sex.
   d. Feelings of intimacy still involved with same sex.
   e. If erotic needs and intimacy needs are not separated - orientation is homosexual.

6. Late adolescence: Begins when satisfactory pattern of sexual behavior is attained:
   a. Self-system becomes stabilized.
   b. Stronger security measures are established to protect from anxiety.
   c. Education and emphasis on society, politics, humanity, the world.

7. Adulthood: Interpersonal relationships finally succeed in changing the animal baby into the human adult.

E. ERIKSON

Erikson's theory of development is a combination of the biological elements from Freud and the social influences of Sullivan. Erikson added to Freud's stages and also was the first theorist to include adulthood as a stage of growth.

For each stage there are problems to be solved and attitudes and abilities to be developed. The conflicts and problems of each stage are never completely resolved and residues are carried forward to be dealt with again at a later stage. The outcomes of each stage can be positive or negative and either outcome affects the identity or the self throughout life. Identity problems involve unsolved problems from any or all other stages. The eight stages of development are:

1. Basic trust versus basic mistrust:
   a. Oral stage.
   b. Consistent and loving care help develop trust.
   c. Inconsistent or harsh care help develop mistrust.
   d. Some mistrust remains in every adult.
2. Autonomy versus shame and doubt:
   a. Anal stage.
   b. Wants to control own thoughts and actions.
   c. Given enough successful choices he feels he can control his body and his environment.
   d. Given enough choices that fail he feels doubt and shame in his own ability to be in charge.
3. Initiative versus guilt:
   a. Oedipal stage.
   b. Explores world with senses, thoughts, and imagination.
   c. Conscience develops helping initiative.
   d. Love relationships with parents, if unsuccessful, lead to feelings of guilt.
4. Industry versus inferiority:
   a. Latency stage.
   b. Understands rules.
   c. Able to work and produce, finish jobs as well as start them.
   d. Inability to satisfy family expectations leads to feelings of inferiority.
5. Identity versus role diffusion:
   a. Genital stage.

b. Rework problems of earlier stages.
c. Seek partner of opposite sex.
d. Attempt to integrate his past and present roles, his body concept with reality, his identity and place in society.

6. Intimacy versus isolation:
   a. Sense of identity necessary to establish intimacy.
   b. Intimacy involves commitment to specific relationship and abiding by the commitment.
   c. Understanding others and letting others understand him.
   d. Isolation results when intimacy is never attained.

7. Generativity versus self-absorption:
   a. Development of next generation.
   b. Includes creativity as well as procreativity.
   c. Without concern for next generation and future generation an individual becomes absorbed in self and stagnates.

8. Ego integrity versus despair:
   a. Integrity results when an individual is satisfied with own actions and life style.
   b. Feels life is meaningful.
   c. Optimistic and still growing.
   d. Failures, and feeling that it is too late to change, lead to despair.

J. PIAGET

Only Piaget among the theorists was concerned with development of cognition. Whereas Freud evolved a theory of childhood development by studying adults, Piaget studied children.

Children learn through imitation and play. Both of these activities demonstrate the dual process of assimilation and accommodation. During assimilation, external or environmental stimuli are altered to fit the schema while during accommodation the schema adjusts to the stimuli. These processes are usually in some degree of temporary balance but accommodation is more apparent during imitation and assimilation during play.

Schemas are patterns of actions or thoughts which form a structural framework for processing and adapting to new incoming data. The structure is constantly altered by the continuous action of the functional processes. The functions of assimilation and accommodation are permanent throughout the developmental period, but structures are temporary. If they were not, development could not occur.

Cognitive development consists of integrating the previous structure into new and more complex behavior patterns. The structure is organized into units called stages. Each stage builds upon the stage before, reorganizing and adapting. Progress through the various stages is linear and, whether fast or slow, proceeds through the stages in order. Progress is affected by individual differences and social influences. The stages number four (with many substages along the way):

1. Sensorimotor:
   a. From birth until about two.
   b. Without language.
   c. Learning relationships with external objects.
   d. Discovers an object is permanent and exists even when not visible.
   e. At first all actions are physical.
   f. Slowly develops ability to "think" and to use language.
   g. Learns to control body in space.
2. Preoperational:
   a. About 2-7 years of age.
   b. Learns to use symbols.
   c. Learns to imitate, to play.
   d. Egocentric - understands only his own viewpoint.
   e. Animistic thinking - inanimate objects have powers and abilities.
3. Concrete operations:
   a. About 7-11 years of age.
   b. Can think and deal with objects and relationships that are visible.
   c. Not egocentric. Feels his own reasoning should agree with the reasoning of others.
   d. More socialized and rule conscious.
   e. Beginning to understand cause and effect in concrete situations.
   f. Knows that changing the shape of objects doesn't change amount, weight, volume, or number.
4. Formal operations:
   a. About 11-15 years of age.
   b. Thinks and reasons in purely abstract terms.
   c. Makes and tests hypotheses.
   d. Thinks logically and sees possibilities.
   e. Difficulty reconciling idealistic hopes with practical possibilities.
   f. Once again egocentric.

When a child has developed his abstract thinking to its fullest he is capable of all the mental operations needed by the adult.

No new structures occur after adolescence. Unlike the other theorists, Piaget's theory does not suggest that the adult is in any way reworking or adapting previous stages and problems.

There is no way to skip a Piagetian stage completely. Abstract thinking cannot be developed without successfully mastering concrete operations. The same situation exists with the other stages.

SUMMARY OF DEVELOPMENTAL THEORIES

Although all four theorists feel that no stage is ever completely replaced by a later one, Piaget does state that no stage can occur until the previous one has been completed. The Freudian adult has oral, anal, phallic, latent and genital traits. The Sullivanian adult still has "enemies", may see himself as "good-bad me" and uses parataxic communication. The Eriksonian adult feels mistrust, guilt, and shame, is creative, industrious, and still has identity problems. The Piagetian adult may sometimes think concretely and have trouble seeing things from another point of view, but if he has not learned to deal with visible objects and relationships, and cannot understand cause and effect, he will not be thinking abstractly.

Both Freud and Sullivan, developed their theories while working with pathological subjects and continued to stress pathology, anxiety, unconscious and uncontrollable drives: an ego or self-system constantly in need of defending. Erikson emphasized both health and illness in the personality, the manageable problems to be solved, and the "identity" which integrates the individual and society. Piaget dealt with normal children and stressed the cognitive development in nonpathological children, the cognitive tasks to be actively accomplished, and the process of learning.

Piaget acknowledged that development was influenced by individual differences and social influences but focused on mind rather than self. Freud considered the early feelings and experiences repressed in the unconscious mind as the causative factor in later neuroses. Sullivan agreed with the unconscious mind concept but focused upon the function of interpersonal relationships as affecting pathological development. Erikson used psychoanalytic concepts combined with the social forces of the larger society.

Without understanding the content and meanings of the patient's unconscious, Freud felt no change in behavior or improvement could be effected. Sullivan assumed that improving interpersonal relationships combined with understanding of basic good-bad transformations could effect change. Erikson integrated aptitudes, libido, and social roles to effect behavioral change and a stronger ego-identity. Piaget thought socialization processes could facilitate cognitive development.

Only Piaget did not emphasize ego, anxiety, identity, libido, or other psychoanalytic concepts. All four considered symbols and communication but Piaget did so with the abstract-concrete thinking of "normal" individuals, Sullivan with the schizophrenic pathological distortions, and Erikson with the more sociopathic manifestations of adolescent character problems.

Freud, Sullivan, and Erikson's theories have been considered universally applicable at some time in their histories; Piaget's theory was ignored for 40 years and is still often considered to be applicable to a select group of upper-class European children. In recent years, Piaget has become more popular and the others less popular.

Freud is still the most widely known of the theorists possibly because he has always stressed the psychosexual aspects of development. Sullivan and Erikson emphasized psychosocial aspects and Piaget focused on the cognitive-interactive aspects.

For Freud, the three stages completed before five years of age influenced all later neurotic behavior and few changes were possible after this age. He especially stressed the role of unresolved Oedipal and/or castration conflicts in later neuroses. Freud saw sexual problems as the basis for aberrant behavior. Sullivan saw sexual problems as just one type of faulty interpersonal relationship affecting behavior and change was usually possible with improved relationships. Erikson viewed change as not only possible but to be expected throughout life and saw sexual identity as one of many problems solvable by the interaction of individual desire and social process. Piaget considered sex to be a variable affecting learning (with age, I.Q., etc.) and expected little change in the adult cognitive structure after middle adolescence.

Although only Piaget worked solely with children, each of the theorists seemed to stress one age as more important or worked with one age group more than the others did.

Freud focused on the first five years of life, Piaget on the middle years of childhood, Sullivan defined three different stages of adolescence, and Erikson alone dealt with middle age and the elderly. Piaget focused on cognitive (including psychomotor) skills, Freud on emotional development, Sullivan on emotional and interpersonal, and Erikson on emotional, interpersonal, and spiritual. Together they encompassed all of man from birth to death, as self or socialized being, while defining psychomotor, emotional, social and cognitive development. They differ in emphasis and direction but each theorist stresses childhood development as a most influential force in adult behavior.

DEVELOPMENTAL THEORIES AND NURSING

If all behavior has meaning, if childhood development influences adult behavior, if nursing process includes planning and evaluating behavioral changes - then developmental theory is a basic frame of reference for making nursing observations and for planning nursing care.

A patient's emotional functioning is a product of his development, his interpersonal relationships, and his immediate stresses. He does not always function adequately, productively, or appropriately. A knowledge and understanding of developmental stages enables a nurse to identify behaviors which demonstrate a malfunction or gap in the growth pattern, to recognize the structural weaknesses, and to help the patient compensate.

The psychiatric nurse will find some behaviors totally unacceptable. Understanding the meanings of such behaviors enables the nurse to intervene more effectively to help the patient modify them.

Pathological behaviors differ from "normal" behaviors only in degree and/or timing. Behavior appropriate at the age of two is not adequate at the age of forty. An adolescent may be a great athlete or actress in fantasy but if he thinks he's Christ or Napoleon and acts accordingly, he has a problem. Group membership may include a vocabulary understood only by the group - a private, secret form of communication to exclude outsiders, but schizophrenic communication excludes other schizophrenics as well as outsiders and may leave the individual unable to communicate effectively with anyone.

The nurse meets the patient "where he is" at the moment, with the goal of changing where he is, of helping him to move towards growth. Yet giving information on an abstract level to a patient who can relate only to concrete details is self-defeating. People who are ill or anxious tend to become more concrete and trying to think abstractly becomes a task that is frustrating to both patient and nurse.

The nurse meets the patient "where he is" in development. It is a waste of time to give information in abstract terms to a patient who can handle only concrete details. Any attempt to treat a 20-year-old patient as 20 years old when he is functioning on a 5-year-old level frustrates both nurse and patient.

No one expects a patient to stand unsupported if he has lost a leg. Why expect him to function without support when he has lost his sense of identity, his self-esteem, his cognitive abilities? But the man with one leg is not totally incapacitated and neither is the man with a loss of identity. Rarely is a psychiatric patient located at the extreme right end of the wellness-illness continuum. Usually there are healthy aspects with which to work in planning interventions and these aspects need to be emphasized - not the aspects of malfunctioning or of deficiency.

REVIEW QUESTIONS

1. What are the developmental stages as defined by Freud? Sullivan? Erikson? Piaget?
2. Which theory is most useful in nursing?
3. What are the dynamics of personality as described by Freud?
4. How does the oral individual behave as an adult? The anal? The phallic?
5. What is an Oedipus Complex?
6. What stage would be represented by organized crime? Sigma Theta Tau? ANA?
7. What is parataxic communication?
8. What are the similarities between Freud and Erikson?
9. What is the difference between concrete and abstract thinking?
10. What is animistic thinking?
11. How can you use these theories in psychiatric nursing?

SUGGESTED REFERENCES

1. Anthony, E.J.: "The Significance of Jean Piaget for Child Psychiatry", Br J Med Psychol 29:29-34, 1956

2. Baldwin, A.L.: Theories of Child Development, John Wiley & Sons, Inc., New York, 1968

3. Bischoff, L.J.: Interpreting Personality Theories, Harper & Row, New York, 1964

4. Eckardt, M.H.: "Life is a Juggling Act: Our Concepts of 'Normal' Development - Myth or Reality?", Am J Psychoanal 35: 103-113, No. 3, 1975

5. Engelhart, K.: "Piaget: A Prescriptive Theory for Parents", Maternal-Child Nursing 3:7, Spring, 1974

6. Erikson, E.: Childhood and Society, W.W. Norton & Co., Inc., New York, 1950

7. Erikson, E.: Identity, Youth and Crisis, W.W. Norton & Co., New York, 1968

8. Fraiberg, S.: The Magic Years, Charles Scribner & Sons, 1959

9. Graves, J.D.: "Psychoanalytic Theory: A Critique", Perspectives Psychi Care 11:114-120, No. 3, July-Aug., 1973

10. Hall, C.S. and Gardner, L.: Theories of Personality, John Wiley & Sons, Inc., New York, 1961

11. Hoyman, H.S.: "Models of Human Nature and Their Impact on Health Education", J School Health 44:378-381, No. 7, The American School Health Association, Kent, Ohio, Sept., 1974

12. Leites, N.: The New Ego, Science House, New York, 1971

13. Missildine, W.H.: Your Inner Child of the Past, Simon & Schuster, New York, 1963

14. Modgil, S.: Piagetian Research, Humanities Press, New York, 1974

15. Nars, M.L.: "The Superego and Moral Development in the Theories of Freud and Piaget", Psychoanalytic Study of the Child, International Universities Press, Inc., 1966

16. Payne, D.: The Relationship of Alienation and Piagetian Concepts in Nursing Diabetic Children, University of Florida, Doctoral Dissertation, 1971

17. Phillips, J.L.: The Origins of Intellect Piaget's Theory, W.H. Freeman & Co., San Francisco, 1969

18. Pulaski, M.A.: Understanding Piaget, Harper & Row, New York, 1971

19. Reich, C.A.: The Greening of America, Random House, New York, 1970

20. Rouslin, S.: "Developmental Aggression and its Consequences", Perspectives Psychi Care 4:18, Oct.-Dec., 1975

21. Sullivan, H.S.: The Interpersonal Theory of Psychiatry, W.W. Norton & Co., New York, 1953

22. Vaillant, G.: "Theoretical Hierarchy of Adaptive Ego Mechanisms", <u>Arch Gen Psychi</u> 24:107-118, 1971

PART II: BEHAVIORS AND INTERVENTIONS

CHAPTER 5

THE ANXIOUS PATIENT

OVERT BEHAVIOR

Feelings of anxiety are almost universal in modern society. Anxiety is a defensive reaction to a threatening situation. The symptoms of anxiety are the symptoms of fear: physiological "fight-flight" reactions, worry, panicky feelings, fright. The individual may be afraid of going crazy or of dying. He is restless, has difficulty sleeping. He has difficulty concentrating and his thinking becomes disorganized. An individual may resolve his anxiety normally by:

1. Sublimating unacceptable drives: body contact sports help relieve aggressive urges, painting or gardening satisfy the urge to "make a mess", and pornography relieves a voyeuristic urge.
2. Changing external environmental situations: quitting a tension-filled job, moving away from nagging relatives or in-laws, and divorcing or marrying can change external situations.
3. Changing oneself by developing a more realistic, practical attitude toward problems: realizing that a college program is too difficult and changing, facing the fact that a faltering marriage is worth saving and making positive efforts to save it, admitting that if everyone else is stupid and wrong it probably isn't everyone else - all difficult and rewarding and productive.

If a normal resolution is not possible, the individual may attempt a neurotic resolution without ever facing or knowing what the real issues are. Not being conscious of what the problems are, he may try to "bind" his anxiety, to fix it in some particular area, or to dissociate it from the rest of the personality. He may develop:

1. Somatic neurosis: Sometimes called hypochondriasis. Anxiety is fixed on the body. May try to prove illness is real. Common somatic manifestations are diarrhea, vomiting, tachycardia, insomnia. Many organs or systems may be involved at once.

   Hypochondriasis is not the same as psychophysiologic disorder. In the psychophysiological (or psychosomatic) disorder, only one organ system is primarily involved, there may be functional or structural changes, and they result from the interaction of stress, organ weakness, and personality with an emotional need or "readiness" for action to relieve tension. Common psychophysiological disorders are ulcers, colitis, hypertension, asthma, obesity.
2. Symbolic neuroses: Anxiety is transformed into bizarre behavior:
   a. Phobias: Anxiety bound up in fear of a particular object or situation (cats, blood, elevators). Experiences terror and uncontrollable apprehension when confronted with phobic ob-

ject. Phobias tend to spread to other objects and may make a prisoner of the individual who is afraid to leave his home for fear he will meet the dreaded object.

b. Conversion hysteria: Anxiety expressed in special kinds of physical symptoms occurring only in body functions which are under the voluntary control (muscles) or conscious interpretation (senses) of the patient, although the symptoms (paralysis, hysterical blindness) may mimic central nervous system problems.

c. A companion to conversion is dissociative hysteria in which anxiety is expressed in defects of memory and awareness. The patient dissociates himself from his past, his surroundings, himself, as a means of flight from danger or crisis. In amnesia he forgets some or all of the past; in fugue he travels long distances without knowing how or why; in multiple personality states he slips from one personality to another.

d. Obsessive-compulsive neurosis: Anxiety is bound up in persistent painful ideas (obsession) or in repetitive, ritualistic, physical acts (compulsion). The obsessive patient fears that his obsessions may occur and has no desire to carry them out. The compulsive patient needs to carry out his compulsions and fears they may be interfered with. The obsessive-compulsive patient uses compulsive behavior to "control" his obsessions. Obsessive-compulsive behavior may become totally incapacitating (complex rituals may interfere with eating, sleeping, functioning) or self-destructive (self-mutilation).

PSYCHODYNAMICS

The ego tries to maintain harmony between the Id and superego impulses within and harmony between the individual and the world outside.

Ordinarily the balance is maintained by gratifying Id impulses, sublimating them, or repressing them. When the balance is threatened, anxiety arises as a signal of danger to the ego.

Repression is an automatic process. Impulses or thoughts unacceptable to the ego are denied, shut off from conscious awareness, and "buried" in the unconscious. The repressed materials remain charged with feeling. If the repressed data are stimulated or the ego weakened, the balance between that which is repressed and the repressing ego is threatened and symptoms of anxiety appear. The purpose of neurotic symptoms is to:

1. Intensify the defense of the repressed, or
2. Allow some of the repressed to come through in symbolic form.

Although all the neurotic reactions due to anxiety reflect similar dynamics, there are some differences in behavior. Since all behavior has meaning and all behavior is purposeful, behavior can illustrate difference in dynamics.

1. Somatic neurosis: When an illness serves a purpose (missing school, avoiding a stressful job, being taken care of) the symptom may well be an expression of anxiety. Behavior patterns appropriate in infancy prove ineffective at a later stage. The regressive needs (total dependency, family structure of childhood, instant gratification) are inappropriate and this is the basic disorder. Behaviors reflect the oral stage of development. Primary defense mechanism: regression.

2. Symbolic neurosis:
   a. Phobia: Focus of phobia must be avoided even if such avoidance leads to violent destructive behavior. May function well when not confronted with specific phobia. A phobia object may symbolize different conflicts in different people and the conflict cannot be deduced from the phobia alone. Conflict may be sexual and arise during phallic stage, symbolism is parataxic in nature and thinking is somewhat animistic. Primary defense mechanism: displacement.
   b. Conversion: Conflict is often sexual in nature (Oedipal or "primal scene") and symptoms prevent acting-out the repressed desires. May serve as either a defense against the repressed or a distorted expression of the repressed. Primary defense mechanism: conversion.
   c. Dissociative hysteria: the patient flees to avoid his conflicts. He becomes not physically unable to act-out but unable to do the forbidden by reason of forgetting it, being geographically removed from it, or by becoming another personality. Primary defense mechanism: dissociation.
   d. Obsessive-compulsive neurosis: Conflict involves hostile-aggressive impulses more than sexual. In an effort to protect the self from destruction by others he displays rigid restricted behaviors of the anal stage and an overdeveloped superego can both express the repressed and punish for the expression. Primary defense mechanism: obsessive-reaction formation, compulsive-undoing.

The phobic patient converts his conflict into external situations which can be avoided. The conversion patient converts his conflict into somatic symptoms which prevent his acting on the repressed wish. The dissociative converts his conflicts into physical or mental flight to prevent his acting-out the repressed. The obsessive-compulsive patient converts his conflict into an elaborate system of rituals so that he can "actively" deal with the repressed or into recurring thoughts that advise him to avoid acting-out the repressed.

Example: Desire to touch or manipulate genitalia of someone close.

1. Phobic: develops fear of all phallic symbols, of closed spaces, of open spaces, soon is confined to own home and away from temptation.
2. Conversion: arm(s) become paralyzed, unable to use hand, no organic cause.
3. Dissociative: finds himself in a distant town, cannot remember traveling or why he traveled, is effectively removed from temptation.

4. Obsessive-compulsion: washes hands frequently, always keeps at least two chairs between self and anyone else, always walks around the chair three times before sitting down, or may have persistent thoughts of having contracted VD or having become pregnant.

Example: Desire to kill or harm someone:

1. Phobic: fear of all weapons, blood, cemeteries, open spaces, people. Unable to act.
2. Conversion: blindness, paralysis, seizures. Unable to see or act.
3. Dissociative: forgets the past - no longer a reason to act.
4. Obsessive-compulsive: frequent thoughts of killing someone other than desired target, self-mutilation, constant washing, may become obedient and willing servant to the target, always takes off the left shoe before the right, always wears clean white gloves, etc.

NURSING INTERVENTION

Nursing interventions are supportive in nature. The neurotic manifestations are inhibiting and unpleasant. Neurotic symptoms may make an individual comfortable for the moment, but comfortable isn't well. Frequently the person has more than one neurotic manifestation (phobias, obsessions, compulsions) resulting in a painful life style.

Protect the phobic patient from his fears, the obsessive-compulsive from interference with rituals.

The anxious patient needs his symptom. However, secondary gain from his symptom may well interfere with the patient's movement towards health.

Reassurance is helpful for the anxious individual. To be able to display neurotic symptoms without fear of being stripped of his defenses may give him the strength to look at his behavior. Once he can view his behavior he may be able to begin identifying purposes.

Unless the patient can develop enough courage and insight to view his symptoms as inhibiting, he may be unwilling to give them up. They may be inefficient but they are the only defenses available at the moment.

Sometimes a patient can give up his symptoms by accepting and understanding his inhibitions even though he can't control them. Factual information may help him.

Obsessive-compulsive behavior is difficult to deal with. He is so intolerant of and unwilling to accept his repressed attitudes and feelings that it is hard for him to cooperate with anyone who wishes to help him change his self-defeating behavior.

The ritualistic individual is very trying and frustrating. The nurse's own anxiety and unresolved problems from the anal stage may interfere with her performance. As in any interpersonal situation, it is important for the nurse to identify her own feelings.

The anxious patient needs to maintain his physical health. Vomiting, fear of dishes or food, rituals that prevent sleep or rest, paralysis may all interfere with the patient's physical maintenance system.

Close observation is needed to identify behaviors, plan care, and intervene successfully. Communication will facilitate interpersonal relations with the patient and help maintain continuity of care.

Because of the frustrating anxiety-provoking behavior displayed in neurotic symptoms, many of the nursing staff take turns working with them. The greater number of staff involved with any patient increases the validity and reliability of the observations and the need for accurate communication.

The intervention procedure recommended when intervening in anxiety hinges on the nurse's ability to <u>first</u> recognize the patient's anxiety.

The steps are to help the patient to:

1. Recognize his anxiety, look at his feelings.
2. Gain insight and new ways of dealing with the threat.
3. Recognize how he is manifesting anxiety in his behavior.
4. Re-evaluate the threat.
5. See the real cause of his distress.
6. Help the patient to see the threat to which he is reacting.
                        (Anxiety, Programmed Text)

Although nursing intervention needs to be individualized for any anxious patient, some approaches are appropriate in ordinary situations. The nurse can:

1. Be supportive and accepting: doesn't respond emotionally to the patient's behavior; doesn't pass judgment on the patient; tries to understand the patient's feelings and behaviors and validates interpretations with the patient; adjust to the patient's overt behavior; set limits when necessary.
2. Try to relieve stress or satisfy need as quickly as possible: remove a phobic patient from the phobic object or the object from the patient; doesn't interfere with compulsive rituals; doesn't push the methodical compulsive or restrain the phobic.
3. Identify patients at oral, anal, or phallic developmental stages and proceed accordingly: the patient with unsatisfied oral needs functions at a regressed infantile level of behavior, is impatient, demanding, dependent and constantly seeking reassurance. They need to have these needs met (in varying degrees) before they can become more independent and self-assured.

    The patient with unsatisfied anal needs functions at a regressed level of behavior also, is neat, finicky, precise, and has difficulty with authority. They need help in maintaining control of themselves and their lives, limitless time for a given task and physical care when their rituals (handwashing, delaying bedtime) endanger their health.

The patient with unresolved sexual conflicts arising during the phallic stage functions on a less noticeably regressed level and is often viewed as immature or adolescent. He is attention-seeking, emotionally labile, and ambivalent in feelings toward the opposite sex. Suggestion is most effective in dealing with "hysterical" patients (but is not used with other anxious patients). Since there may also be a problem with latent homosexuality, physical contact is kept to a minimum when the patient's display of anxiety warrants this.

4. Listen: ask any patient
5. Protect his defenses: he has no other defense. Leave him his rituals, respect his phobia, care for his blindness - while helping him identify his behaviors.
6. Encourage the patient's self-expression, verbal or concrete: sometimes talking can relieve or lessen the need for the neurotic behaviors; activities can replace rituals.
7. Identify own feelings: sometimes an unresolved conflict in a patient triggers the same unresolved conflict in the nurse and leads to a destructive circular behavior pattern in which each reinforces the other's pathology and neither can break the circle. Understanding her own conflict is not necessary for intervening and halting the nontherapeutic relationship. Identifying the feelings the patient arouses can afford insight into the behavioral responses and provide a means of altering the relational process. A supervisor or other observant professional may help the nurse look at the nurse-patient relationship and identify feelings and behaviors adversely affecting it. If the conflict becomes pathological, psychiatric assistance can afford further insight and self-understanding.

If the nurse cannot identify the dynamics of the nurse-patient interaction, recognize feelings of anger, guilt, fear, or anxiety then the relationship will be affected and the patient will be forced to deal with the nurse's feelings instead of the nurse dealing with the patient's.

A nurse may have a strong unrecognized need to control people and situations. She will push too fast and unconsciously insist upon the patient's improvement. If the patient can't respond, the nurse may become aggressive and hostile or may withdraw from the relationship. These behaviors confuse a patient and are nontherapeutic.

Nurses are people and have the same conflicts as other people. One conflict the nurse often refuses to face is a sexual conflict. A nurse who doesn't recognize her latent homosexuality may be thrown into an unrecognized panic by an overt homosexual patient, and be unable to identify her behavior. (It's not wise for others to identify her behavior unless appropriate interventions are possible and professional help is available). A nurse who doesn't recognize an unresolved Oedipal conflict may not be able to establish a therapeutic nurse-patient relationship with older male or older female patients.

A nurse who is unable to identify and understand her feelings is always in danger of becoming emotionally involved with a patient. If the involvement is recognized by the patient, perhaps no harm will be done. If the patient does not recognize the nurse's involvement, he may receive two messages in every instruction and not be able to separate the nurse's behaviors as a nurse from her conflicting behaviors as a woman. This is a nontherapeutic relationship that cannot help either the patient or the nurse.

To give effective nursing care the nurse needs to understand the behaviors and developmental stages of the patients. She also needs to understand her own.

REVIEW QUESTIONS

1. How can anxiety by resolved?
2. What happens when anxiety is not resolved?
3. What is a somatic neurosis?
4. What are the types of symbolic neuroses?
5. What are the psychodynamics of anxiety?
6. How do the dynamics of anxiety differ in the somatic and symbolic neuroses?
7. What nursing interventions are appropriate in anxiety?
8. How can the nurse help a phobic patient?
9. What nursing interventions are appropriate in somatic neurosis?

SUGGESTED REFERENCES

1. Anxiety: Recognition and intervention, Programmed instruction, Am J Nursing LXV, Sept., 1965

2. Arietti, S.: The Intrapsychic Self, Basic Books, Inc., New York, 1967

3. Compton, A.: A study of the psychoanalytic theory of anxiety, II, Developments in theory of anxiety since 1926, J Am Psychoanalytic Assoc XX:341-394, 1972

4. Fenichel, O.: The Psychoanalytic Theory of Neuroses, W.W. Norton & Co., New York, 1945

5. Gaarder, K.: Control of states of consciousness, Arch Gen Psychi XXV:436-441, 1971

6. Gelfman, M.: The role of irresponsibility in obsessive-compulsive neuroses, Intervention J Psychi, pp. 36-47, 1970

7. Greenberg, S.: Neurosis is a Painful Style of Life, Signet, The New American Library, New York, 1970

8. Hodgson, R., et al.: The treatment of obsessive compulsive neurosis: Follow-up and further findings, Behavior Research Therapy X:181-189, 1972

9. Horney, K.: The Neurotic Personality of Our Time, W.W. Norton Co., Inc., New York, 1937

10. Horney, K.: Self Analysis, W.W. Norton Co., Inc., New York, 1942

11. Jourard, S.M.: Self-Disclosure, John Wiley & Sons, Inc., New York, 1971

12. Ladar, M.: The nature of anxiety, Br J Psychi CXXI:481-491, 1972

13. MacKenzie, K.R.: The eclectic approach to the treatment of phobias, Am J Psychi CXXX:1103-1106, 1973

14. Maslow, A.H.: The Farther Reaches of Human Nature, The Viking Press, New York, 1971

15. May, R.: Man's Search for Himself, W.W. Norton Co., Inc., 1953

16. May, R.: The Meaning of Anxiety, Ronald Press, New York, 1950

17. Oberst, M.: The crisis-prone staff nurse, Am J Nursing LXXIII:1917-1921, 1973

18. Olson, L.Q.: Intervention in a pathological cycle of anxiety, J Psychi Nursing Mental Health Services XII:21-25, March-April, 1974

19. Pasquali, E.A.: Personification: Patient and nurse problems, Perspectives Psychi Care XIII:58-61, 1975

20. Shapiro, D.: Neurotic Styles, Basic Books, New York, 1965

21. Stringer, M.: Therapeutic nursing intervention following derrogation of the nurse by the patient, Perspectives Psychi Care III:36, 1965

22. Wahl, C.W.: Commonly neglected psychosomatic syndromes, American Handbook of Psychiatry, Arieti, S., Ed., Basic Books, Inc., New York, Vol. III, pp. 158-165, 1966

23. Wahl, C.W.: The techniques of brief psychotherapy with hospitalized psychosomatic patients, International J Psychoanalytic Psychother I:69-82, Nov., 1975

24. Willner, G.: The role of anxiety in obsessive-compulsive disorders, Am J Psychoanal XXVIII:201-211, 1968

CHAPTER 6

THE DEPRESSED PATIENT

It is not always easy to distinguish between what is "normal" and what is neurotic, or what is neurotic and what is psychotic.

If the problems, in whatever form, are related to environmental stresses or sudden losses, the behavior is more neurotic. Much of the energy is wasted on symptoms and diverted from effective, realistic interaction with the world.

The neurotic individual is in contact with reality however, and differentiates symptoms from reality, and can understand and communicate with others.

In psychoses, the disorganization is more complete. The energy is turned inward and focused on the internal conflicts. The psychotic individual has difficulty relating to other people, in differentiating symptom from reality, and in communicating with others. He interprets his symptoms - and the world - differently than do the therapists working with him. The resultant gulf makes treatment difficult.

Quantitatively, the psychotic individual is more bound up in a morbid process than is the neurotic. Qualitatively, he views his symptoms differently. The neurotic individual judges his symptoms according to reality; the psychotic individual judges reality according to his symptoms.

The person with a psychosis does not recognize or acknowledge symptoms. The symptom becomes reality, and reality itself is distorted to fit the symptom.

Depression is a normal affect, a natural emotion we can all experience and suffer from. It can be placed on a continuum from normal to pathological: from sadness, grief, mourning and melancholia to neurotic and manic depressive psychotic diseases. Neurotic depressions frequently occur in combination with other neurotic symptoms, such as anxiety and hysteria; psychotic depressions are classified as manic depressive, schizoaffective, involutional, and postpartum psychoses.

Depression spans the ages, beginning with anaclitic depressions of infancy and early childhood. Depression frequently combines and masks anxiety to cause hyperactivity in the school-aged child. Neurotic depressions, like other neurosis, occur most frequently between the ages of 20 and 40, while involutional melancholia occurs at climacteria and disengagement depressions are seen in the aged.

While most depressions tend to be time bound and self-limiting, manic depressive psychoses reoccur cyclically and six or seven brief hospitalizations are not uncommon in the afflicted person's life span.

Three etiologically significant areas explain depression: the analytic syndrome, the genetic and the biochemical hypothesis. The practitioner needs to be aware of the components of these explanations, since nurses frequently encounter depressed persons in practice and the accurate assessment of lethality can be a life-saving measure (see Appendix A). Often the depressed person is not aware of his psychological symptoms and seeks medical help for the physical manifestations of the emotion. The threat of suicide in depression is its most formidable outcome. One study found 50 percent of the patients had made office visits to clinics seeking treatment of their physical symptoms the week preceding their suicide (Coppen). This is tragic, since once diagnosed, the treatment of depressions is usually successful, alleviating the patient's burdensome pain. In the last decade, the most significant biological research findings in the psychiatric area have been the expansion of knowledge in treatment of depressions (Brodie, 1975).

SADNESS, GRIEF, AND MOURNING

Sadness and grief are normal emotional and physical adaptive reactions to any personal loss of consequence: changes in home or jobs, body image, emotional detachment from significant relationships, as through death of a loved one, separation from a dear friend, divorce, or maturation and individuation of children (empty nest syndrome). Changes in the person's life and in the person's behavior are significant. If the grief is in response to awareness of serious or fatal illness, the grief may interfere with the treatment even though the grief responses are realistic.

The "loss complex" may seem exaggerated or inappropriate to the observer. The loss may have personal intrapsychic meanings, symbolically tied to the individual's past with special, catastrophic meanings that are unrelated to reality. These trigger a depression because of the individual's unique frame of reference. The loss may be associated with guilt feelings and the person becomes "numb" because it is too painful to grieve - too painful to feel. Often there are ambivalent feelings about the person who has died or the personal loss. Over-endowed with symbolic meaning, feelings of hate stimulate guilt when "love" is expected of self.

The painful guilt that is stimulated often is "dissociated". The popular notion is that to experience sadness or show emotion is a sign of weakness and "stiff upperlipmanship" is applauded. It is often said someone "took it well", inferring that blocked dissociations of feelings are a sign of strength. Conversely, the nurse often encounters persons in times of crisis and loss who are nonreactive and devoid of the emotional expressions the nurse "expects". Often nature provides patients and families a defense so they can go about their business and preserves their limited energies for doing what must be done. During these times, people need support for their lack of feelings so they do not conjure up self-derogatory self-concepts of being "cold" or "unfeeling". The nurse's approach should be to sustain the patient in his experiences; it is counterproductive to encourage him to cry or produce emotions unconsciously walled-off. Also, since he is unable to feel, having dissociated the feelings outside awareness, expecting or asking him to respond merely increases the guilt often found in grief reactions. The nurse should avoid paving the way for depression instead of sustaining him in his impending grief (Ujhely, 1966).

Health care workers have a tendency to avoid persons experiencing grief for a variety of reasons:

1. It is painful to witness distress in another human.
2. Seeing tears and other signs of "letting go", they fear what's next and doubt they can handle it.
3. If related to medical or nursing management, the person often expresses anger and resentment toward the therapist.
4. The therapist may have unresolved grief and this is painfully reawakened by empathic responses.
5. The therapist feels helpless and is unaware that listening is doing something.

GRIEF WORK

Successful resolution of grief is essential, if a person is unable to experience sadness, he may become depressed. Depression can be viewed as a defense against sadness. If not experienced, held in abeyance, the person is left without integration of the loss. Unresolved grief leaves something painfully disturbing in people; there is a residual distortive adaptation and a constant drain on their energies as they strive to keep the feeling of sadness repressed. Additional losses later in life may trigger the unresolved grief of the earlier losses, as do "anniversary" reactions. To sustain the patient in his subjective experience so the loss can be integrated in his life stream and he can grow, the following nursing approaches are suggested:

1. Employ anticipatory guidance prior to losses when they can be predicted. Guiding parents as children mature and "move on", preoperative education and exploration of changes in body image in scheduled mutilating surgery.
2. Elicit inferred feelings of loss with statements as "you seem to be hurting emotionally".
3. Assist the patient in acknowledging feelings cognitively and viscerally, unifying the somatic components of emotional response.
4. Accept the specific meaning of the loss to the patient providing a safe, accepting environment for him to talk.
5. Learn to tolerate intensity of feelings, knowing they will proceed in a natural course.
6. Provide the patient opportunities to express feelings by crying, or through clarifying physical symptoms as chest pains, head and visceral disturbances.
7. Anticipate previous losses, "unfinished business" will also require rehashing, grieving, and resolution.

Grief work cannot be hurried; its time and depth varies among individuals. Often, in the process of accepting one's loss, the person retreats from reality and clings to the past. There is a withdrawal of interest in others, as grief work requires the expenditure of energy and time on self. Memories must be painfully re-experienced as the person is forced to acknowledge past investments are no longer available. There is a mobilization of contradictory feelings, especially when the loss represents a wish-fulfillment on an unconscious level. There is anger, both inwardly and outwardly expressed, a loss of usual conduct patterns, and often the "taking on" of characteristics of the lost person. There may be somatic problems as the person moves to gradually accept reality. Grief work is a process with sequential steps through which the person must painfully progress to accommodate to loss and reality, and adjust to the changed; otherwise, there is a fleeing to defensive depression and possible mental illness. The steps in grief work are (Kubler-Ross, 1969):

1. Denial and isolation
2. Anger
3. Bargaining
4. Depression
5. Acceptance and hope

Some support a biochemical etiological explanation of depression, based on two serendipitous drug reactions introduced by physical medicine in the mid-fifties. Reserpine, used in the treatment of hypertension, had as a side effect severe clinical depression with an appreciable suicide rate. Neuropharmacological studies showed reserpine depleted norepinephrine, serotonin and dopamine from the brain. The second group of drugs, monoamine oxidase inhibitors, were used to treat tuberculosis. These were found to have euphoric side effects. Their use was extended to antidepressants for the treatment of depression. MAO inhibitors increased the biogenic amines (dopamine, norepinephrine and serotonin) in the brain. These findings led to later research exploring the possibility that an alteration in biogenic amine metabolism might be the pathophysiological basis of depressive disorders.

Adding to diagnostic complexity of depressions is the fact that depression and organic diseases may co-exist. For example, depression is seen early in the course of carcinoma of the pancreas before somatic symptoms appear. Depression secondary to organic illness does not minimize the importance of treatment of depression and the physical problems concurrently.

Genetic research shows a positive family history in psychotic depressions. However, the suggestability of neurotics and their tendency to resolve problems through imitation and example provided the rationale for providing survivors of suicides therapeutic support. The "psychological autopsy" is a useful therapeutic tool since survivors are usually left a sequelae of unresolved emotional turmoil, and become high-risk groups more likely to commit suicide than people from families with no history of suicide (Murphy).

Theories relating depression to endocrine imbalances stress the occurrence of involutional melancholia at climacteria, postpartum psychoses, and the heightened rate of female suicide attempts during the premenstrual period. Research shows premorbid anal trait personality triad of parsimony, perfectionistic and ritualistic behaviors and precipitating loss lay the groundwork for depressive responses. Since depressions frequently present with a mask of anxiety, differential symptomology is important and the following distinctions can be made:

Depression	Anxiety
Slow speech	Intensified speech rate
Reluctant to talk	Talks eagerly
Monotonous voice	Animated, variable vocal tones
Repetitive, constricted topics	Content varied
Talking doesn't change effect	Suggestible - talking can lead to behavior changes
Lacks interest	Interest circumscribed
Doesn't enjoy things	Can enjoy some things
Worse in morning	Worse in evening
Poor appetite with weight loss	May eat more (except in anorexia nervosa)
Constipated	Diarrhea
Helped by antidepressant	Worsened by antidepressants
Worsened by tranquilizers	Helped by tranquilizers

In distinguishing depression from schizophrenia, the following differences can usually be found:

Depression	Schizophrenia
The therapist feels empathetic toward the behaviours	The therapist is puzzled by the behaviours
Affect and thinking are related	Inappropriate "split" between content and response (as smiling while saying they feel sad)
Blocking of thoughts	Loose associations
History of some stable interpersonal relationships	History of inadequate interpersonal relationships

It isn't a matter of how excessive the reaction appears or how long it lasts. What is important is the attitude of the individual, how he views reality, and how well he can relate to people around him.

Depressions are defined not only as neurotic or psychotic but also as:

1.   - (neurotic or reactive) resulting from external and environmental stimulus.
2. Endogenous - (psychotic) resulting from early personality deficit.

Loss of a love object is a necessary factor in any depression. Loss may sometimes be the precipitating factor in a depressive episode.

Whatever the type or the cause, depression has its own recognizable behaviors and its own dynamics. And whether neurotic or psychotic, understandable or bizarre - the behavior has meaning and purpose for the one displaying it.

OVERT BEHAVIOR

Physiological processes slow down, muscles sag, posture slumps, face appears sad, walk is slow and dragging.

The individual cries often, has difficulty sleeping, loses his appetite. He cannot think well due to both lack of ideas and inability to concentrate.

He loses interest in his physical being, may become constipated, dirty, sick. Whereas the neurotic depressed individual may become more depressed as the day progresses, the psychotic feels lowest in the morning and may improve during the day. However, in a recent research study from England (Stallone) less than 50 percent of the depressed patients had any such diurnal change.

Severe delusional ideation may occur, usually somatically based. The individual may explain his lack of appetite by saying he has no stomach or his bowels have turned into snakes or his mouth is a cave with no exit.

He feels completely worthless, voices this feeling verbally and in his body language. At first he may be ritualistic or hostile; as his depression progresses, he becomes increasingly gloomy. His actions may range from a simple lack of interest in his surroundings to an almost motionless stupor. He is, at one and the same time, indifferent to his environment and sensitive to it.

He may voice thoughts of suicide, of wanting to be left alone to die. He's pessimistic about all outcomes and discourages approaches of others. He often denies any depression.

PSYCHODYNAMICS

One of the functions of the ego is to mediate and maintain a balance between Id and Superego. In depression, there is internal disintegration with "de-fusion" of the instincts as the ego capitulates to the self-punitive superego.

The dynamic elements of depression are:

1. Manipulation (dependency)
2. Aversion to influence
3. Hostility
4. Unwillingness to give gratification
5. Anxiety

The oral traits of the personality are most pronounced. The individual has a great need for reassurance, support, and acceptance from the outside world. He is excessively dependent upon the love, affection, and encouragement given him by others. Without a constant input of "build-up" from the world around him, he feels lost, deserted and angry.

He seems to lack inner resources and strength. Being emotionally greedy, his needs cannot be satisfied by anyone or anything and he is disappointed. He becomes involved in a vicious circular reaction. He demands more from others, they cannot satisfy him, he is disappointed, and demands still more. The more he demands, the more others reject him; the more others reject him the more he demands.

When demands are not met and needs not satisfied, the individual becomes hostile and angry towards those who reject him. Then he feels guilty because of the hostility and develops strongly self-punitive attitudes.

Precipitating factors in a depressive psychosis are those which make increased demands on an oral person, demands which take something from him or ask something of him. He cannot meet the demands and feels angry and frustrated, but his superego won't let him express his hostility directly to the world. He turns the anger in on himself, says, "I'm no good, I've never been any good, I'll never be any good", and punishes himself in his depression.

A recent study comparing Caucasian and Oriental college girls (Marsella) found a discrepancy between the ideal-self and the real-self in depression.

NURSING INTERVENTIONS

Approaching and communicating with a depressed patient is difficult. At first he withdraws. If he feels dependent upon a relationship he will both fight it and seek it, the ambivalence causing more hostility, more guilt, more depression. Certain attitudes are important for the nurse:

1. Honesty - he can't tolerate more disappointment. The nurse needs to be truthful and must not make promises she may not be able to keep.
2. Nonrejection - he receives and gives nothing in return, arousing feelings of irritability and impatience in others. The nurse needs to avoid displaying any behavior which could be interpreted as rejecting or depreciating.
3. Interest - he feels unworthy and a lack of interest reinforces this. When he feels the nurse is not interested but works with him as a "duty", he feels more worthless and more depressed.
4. Empathy - he is depressed by a "cheerful giver". His feelings are real and his depression won't go away if he just "cheers up".
5. Support - he feels he is evil and will taint others. If the nurse can support anyone as unworthy without being injured, he feels perhaps that he is not as worthless as he thought.
6. Acceptance - he is unable to express his feelings, sometimes acts strangely. Unless he can be accepted for what he is, he will not be able to recognize what he is and try to change.

Nursing care varies in degree and emphasis as the patient moves from a deep, withdrawn depression to a more effective functioning condition.

Some areas of nursing care are emphasized more at one time than at another:

1. Communication - even though he may not respond at first, he needs to be talked to, addressed by his name, and listened to. He may be able to manage conversation first on neutral topics, then move on to more personal discussion.

   (Weissman's study indicates that working-class depressed women improved more with supportive therapy than with insight. Talking about present problems was more productive than trying to probe childhood experiences.)

   The nursing approach to the depressed patient provides for an interpersonal experience in communication that loosens the bonded feelings. The steps are:
   a. Brief, frequent conversations on neutral topics to initiate the relationship, accepting that the patient has a low impulse for communication and interpersonal contact.
   b. Gradual establishment of a nonthreatening "safe" environment.
   c. Help the patient become aware of his emotional flatness by direct confrontation.
   d. Calmly accept the denial and angry responses of the patient.
   e. Provide opportunities for the patient to perceive his anger and the nondestructive outcomes when he is able to express anger.
   f. Encourage elaboration and detailed descriptions of past frustrations.
   g. Provide opportunities for him to verbally and emotionally explore past painful grievances.
   h. Assist him in getting congruence in his verbal-nonverbal systems.
   i. Develop strategies to gradually break the bonds by expanding his self-awareness.
   j. Evaluation of effectiveness of approach by the patient's ability to form new attachments and commitments to life outside himself.

   Much body language is spoken in his blank, unexpressive face, the monotonous tone of his voice and his slow, painful movements that lack spontaneity. Even in silence he can "not communicate" (Wozlowick). His actions speak louder than words, conveying his helplessness and anger. The nonverbal messages make the depressed person particularly unpleasant to be around. Others move away in self-protection, or become angered by his impervious veneer. By provoking anger, he further legitimizes his own and the binding web of depression thickens.

   The incongruence between the verbal and nonverbal messages contribute to the "unrealness" of the depressive. Terrified of his feelings, he has cut off awareness of others and himself.

Ruesch (1959) attributes the depressive's anger to a lack of balance between goals and gratification, and compares the mismatch of verbal and nonverbal to the frustration of the aphasic who cannot speak the words that match his thoughts and feelings. The depressive's behavior represents the popularly held misconception that any display of anger is "dangerous"; actually an angry speaking out in ego defense to keep communications lines open and maintain interpersonal interactions is healthy.

The nurse's basic task with a depressed patient is to lessen his feelings of guilt and worthlessness and increase his self-esteem. He needs to be protected from self-harm and physical consequences of his personal apathy and neglect. His activities are planned to increase his communication with others, integrate him into productive relationships and lessen his feelings of hopelessness.

2. Physical care - in depression, physical well-being may be forgotten or the patient may not be capable of caring for himself. The more severe the depression, the more important is physical care.

   a. He needs to have his diet monitored. He is too disinterested or too apathetic to eat. He may feel he is too evil to deserve food. He may need assistance at mealtime as a small child does, or he may actually need to be fed. Intake and output records are helpful in planning care.

   b. His skin may break down from lack of fluids or lack of care. He may need lotions. He may need to be bathed if he cannot bathe himself.

   c. A regular daily rhythm of mood, energy, and ability to function is reported by most depressed patients. Psychotic depressives fall asleep easily, awaken early and feel better as the day progresses; neurotics feel better in the morning, becoming more depressed as the day progresses. The quality of sleep is poor with diminished REM sleep and difficulty falling asleep. His disturbed sleep will affect his recovery. He may need rest periods, a different sleep schedule. On the other hand, he may stay in bed all day without sleeping and needs encouragement to move around. His circulation may be poor and adversely affected by lack of movement.

   d. His appearance is neglected and he may need help in choosing his clothes for the day, and encouragement in dressing and in keeping his clothes washed and pressed. Men may need to be shaved, and women to have their hair done.

3. Protection - suicide is always a real threat with a depressed patient. When he begins to come out of the depression, close observation is still needed, because he may then have the energy and the opportunity to kill himself. He may try "passive" suicide by starvation or falling asleep in the bathtub.

4. Recreation - he needs encouragement to move about and enter into situations with others. Sometimes menial chores help during the worst "unworthy" period, but may be resented later. Such tasks relieve his need for self-condemnation. He feels the lowliest job is what he deserves, yet he receives praise when the job is completed, thus enhancing his self-concept. He feels more worthy when a needed job is done, so simple tasks that can be

finished are effective. The more energy the task requires, the less energy he will have left to direct inward. Team sports use up energy and are also acceptable outlets for aggression and anger.

As is true of any psychiatric patient, the depressed patient's desired change in behavior is accomplished only when he feels some degree of self-esteem, can express his feelings, and has a more realistic self-image and effective life style.

REVIEW QUESTIONS

1. What is the greatest danger facing the depressed patient?
2. What are the dynamics of depression?
3. What are possible preventive measures?
4. How does neurotic depression differ from psychotic depression? How would this affect nursing care?
5. What does the phrase "loss of love object" mean? What meaning does it have in depression?
6. Why is physical care important for the depressed patient?
7. How would nursing care differ in working with a person who was extremely depressed, one who was beginning active therapy, and one who was almost self-sufficient?

SUGGESTED REFERENCES

1. Bonime, W.: On depression, Contemporary Psychoanal XII:49, 1966

2. Brodie, H. and Sabshin, M.: An overview of trends in psychiatric research, Am J Psychi CXXX:1309-1318, 1973

3. Coppen, A.: Depression: A clinical portrait, The Medical Management of Depression, Hill, Sir D. and Hollister, L., Eds., MEDCOM Learning Systems, Lakeside Laboratories, New York, 1970

4. Crory, W.G. and Crory, G.: Depression, Am J Nursing LXXIII: 472-475, March, 1973

5. Davies, B., Ed.: Depressive Illness: Some Research Studies, C.C. Thomas, Springfield, Ill., 1972

6. Drake, R.E.: Depression: Adaptation to disruption and loss, Perspectives Psychi Care VIII:163-170, 1975

7. Flynn, G.: Hostility in a mad mad world, Perspectives Psychi Care IV:148-180, March-April, 1969

8. Foss, G.: Sleep, drugs and dreams, Am J Nursing LXXI:2316-2320, Dec., 1971

9. Freud, S.: Mourning and melancholia, In The Complete Psychological Works of Sigmund Freud, Strachey, Hogart Press, London, Vol. 14, pp. 343-358, 1914-1916

10. Fromm, E.: The Anatomy of Human Destructiveness, Holt, Rinehart & Winston, New York, 1973

11. Hill, F.D.: Nonverbal communication and psychiatric research, Arch Gen Psychi XXVII:631-635, Nov., 1972

12. Kubler-Ross, E.: On Death and Dying, The Macmillan Co., New York, 1969

13. Lewis, A.: "Endogenous" and "exogenous": A useful dichotomy? Psychological Med XI:191-196, 1971

14. Marsella, A.J., et al.: Personality correlates of depressive disorders in female college students of different ethnic groups, International J Social Psychi XVIX:77-81, Spring-Summer, 1973

15. McGraw, R.M.: Grief - its clinical importance and its resolution, Modern Med, pp. 61-65, May, 1972

16. Sattin, S.S.: The psychodynamics of the holiday syndrome, Perspectives Psychi Care XIII:156-163, 1975

17. Murphy, A., et al.: Who calls the suicide prevention center? Am J Psychi CXXVI:314-324, 1969

18. Plath, S.: The Bell Jar, Harper & Row, New York, 1971

19. Pearce, J. and Newton, S.: The Conditions of Human Growth, Citadel Press, New York, pp. 275, 1963

20. Rosenfield, E.M.: Intervening in hostile behavior through dyadic and/or group intervention, J Psychi Nursing Mental Health Nursing, pp. 251-254, Nov.-Dec., 1969

21. Rothenberg, A.: On anger, Am J Psychi CXXVIII:88-96, Oct., 1971

22. Ruesch, J.: Disturbed Communication, W.W. Norton Co., Inc., New York, 1959

23. Sattin, S.M.: The psychodynamics of the holiday syndrome, Perspectives Psychi Care VIII:156-162, 1975

24. Sanborn, D.E. and Sanborn, C.J.: The psychological autopsy as a therapeutic tool, Diseases Nervous System XXXVII:2-8, Jan., 1976

25. Schildkraut, J.J.: Neuropsychopharmacology and the Affective Disorders, Little, Brown & Co., Boston, 1970

26. Shneidman, E.S., et al.: The Psychology of Suicide, Science House, Inc., New York, 1970

27. Spiegel, R.: Anger and acting out, Am J Psychother XXI:597-607, 1967

28. Stallone, F., et al.: Longitudinal studies of diurnal variations in depression, Br J Psychi CXXIII:311-318, Sept., 1973

29. Swanson, A.: Communicating with depressed persons, Perspectives Psychi Care VII, 1975

30. The Quality of Sleep in Depressive Syndromes, Excerpted from a Symposium on Sleep Disorders, sponsored by Pfizer Laboratories Division in Miami, Fla., Nov., 1972

31. Thomas, R.: Anger: A tool for developing self-awareness, Am J Nursing LXX:2586-2589, Dec., 1970

32. Ujhely, G.: Grief and depression: Implication for nursing care, Nursing Forum V:23-35, Feb., 1966

33. Understanding hostility, An Educational Design Program, Programmed Instruction, Am J Nursing LXVII:2131-2149, Oct., 1967

34. Weissman, M. and Klerman, G.: Psychotherapy with depressed women: An empirical study of content themes and reflections, Br J Psychi CXXIII:55-61, July, 1973

35. Williams, T., et al. (Ed.): Recent advances in the Psychobiology of the Depressive Illnesses, Government Printing Office, Washington, D.C., 1972

36. Wozlawick, P., et al.: Pragmatics of Human Communication, W.W. Norton Co., Inc., New York, p. 51, 1967

37. Zung, W.W.K.: Effect of antidepressant drugs on sleeping and dreaming, Biological Psychi I:283-287, 1969

CHAPTER 7

THE ELATED PATIENT

In the manic-depressive psychosis, periods of depression alternate with periods of elation. The dynamics of elation are quite similar to the dynamics of depression. A manic disorder is, in fact, a reaction-formation against depression. However, the behaviors displayed and the nursing interventions required are quite dissimilar.

OVERT BEHAVIOR

Physiological processes are speeded up. Hyperactivity may be extreme enough to endanger life.

Talks loudly and often obscenely. Ideas are expansive; expresses delusions of grandeur. Has short attention span with flight of ideas.

Aggressive and extroverted in behavior. Very distractible and extremely responsive to environmental stimuli.

Has a low frustration tolerance and acts rather than talks. Acting-out behavior may be destructive and dangerous.

Wants everything to be as attractive as possible. Adorns himself with flowers or jewelry, bright clothes, garish combinations. He tries to decorate his surroundings with pictures, paintings, colored cloth, anything colorful and appealing.

Too busy for mundane things, he may forget to eat, eliminate, or sleep. It may be impossible for him to slow down enough to rest.

Meddlesome and domineering, talks constantly, sometimes so fast that he skips words or runs them together.

Love's everyone and tries to incorporate the world. He responds to interference with irritability, hostility and profanity.

Has a keen wit, is observant and sees everything, tries to manipulate others whenever possible.

PSYCHODYNAMICS

As in depression, the ego loses its struggle to mediate the superego and id. This time the ego capitulates to the primitive, pleasure-seeking id. There is the same dependency on external rewards and the same ambivalence toward those who give the rewards. The ego is weakened.

The elated individual feels worthless and useless. Unable to tolerate such feelings, he denies them. The denial leads to anxiety and the superego has to relax, leaving the id in control.

He feels as worthless and useless as the depressed person but responds with arrogance. Being worthless, he feels he doesn't deserve to have his needs met and so, of course, no one will meet them. He sets about manipulating other people to intervene and satisfy his demands. Such manipulation not only protects him from failure, it also gives him a false sense of power and control over those he manipulates.

His demands are excessive and when one person cannot satisfy them, he goes to another and another. As more people reject him, his anxiety increases and he makes more demands.

His elation and hyperactivity is an appeal for love, a protection from depression. He wants to incorporate the world - to love everyone.

NURSING INTERVENTIONS

No matter how aggressive his demands, refusal to meet them rarely leads to a rage reaction.

Setting limits is an important aspect of nursing care for any elated patient. Such external control can give him a greater sense of security, lessen his anxiety, and make him feel that the nurse considers him worth bothering about - just as his mother did.

Any nurse needs self-assurance to set limits without creating a power struggle. The elated patient often argues and needs to receive simple explanations without openings for argument. Demands can be handled in different ways:

1. Postpone satisfaction: His interests change so rapidly, he may forget the demand if satisfaction is postponed.
2. Satisfy: He can't be restricted in everything. May have to have demands met in some areas in order to maintain limits in more important issues.
3. Satisfy part of demand: May be able to cut a grandiose demand to manageable size or to agree to part of it.

When he begins manipulating and playing one member of the treatment team against another:

1. Interrupt the cycle.
2. Identify his manipulative behavior pattern.
3. Maintain group cohesiveness

The elated patient acts out his frustrations instead of discussing them. It is another way to avoid facing problems and may make others avoid him from fear and guilt.

Acting-out is a hostile and controlling act. There must be some responsibility on the patient's part for controlling himself instead of trying to control others. He can learn that acting-out may be caused by fear or frustration and helped to identify his feelings so that he can try to control them.

In the acute acting-out phase, he needs added support and coordinated intervention by the entire health team. Once the acute stage has passed, he can be encouraged to talk it out. The nurse working with an elated patient needs to be:

1. Supportive: his ego can afford him little support and his energies are directed to controlling his depression. The nurse tries to slow him down to accept his elation without entering into his hilarity.
2. Firm yet flexible: the perfectionist nurse may be ineffective with an elated patient for his distractibility, hyperactivity, and inability to concentrate will be difficult to deal with unless the nurse can identify her own feelings of impatience and irritability. The overly-permissive nurse may also be ineffective if she gives the elated patient so little structure that he loses all control.
3. Accepting: he's always testing and will try to persuade other patients or visitors to run errands for him, may annoy other patients and try to "play" one member of the treatment team against another. If the nurse can accept him calmly and intervene decisively, he can be diverted from the undesirable behaviors.
4. Thick-skinned: he can be obscene, insulting, extremely personal and often makes the nurse the brunt of his jokes. Acceptance with decisive firm action can divert him.

The elated patient needs different kinds of nursing care than the depressed patient, although their problem areas may be similar:

1. Communication: Very talkative, needs simple explanations, concise truthful answers to questions - if he waits for an answer. Arguments need to be avoided. Sometimes "laughing with" him helps his integrity, "laughing at" him doesn't.
2. Physical care: He is too busy to eat or take care of himself.
   a. Too busy to eat, too distractible to be able to sit with others, this patient may starve as easily as the depressed patient. He likes "finger foods" that he can eat on the run. Safer for him to be by himself to eat for he is so involved with everyone else he can't concentrate on eating. He also throws things! Intake and output is helpful in planning care. Needs hi-calorie liquids to help prevent his "burning himself out".
   b. His skin may break down from poor nutrition. He perspires a lot and is prone to minor bruises and abrasions.
   c. His sleep is almost nonexistent. His hyperactivity is life-threatening. May die of fatigue, coronary insufficiency, or other related causes. Sometimes sleep can be aided by warm baths, soft music, quiet activities. Extra rest periods or just "quiet times" will help.
   d. His appearance is sometimes unbelievable. Wants to decorate himself with flowers or jewelry, may run around nude. Needs help in selecting his clothes. Difficult to shave men, as they can't sit still. Women wear too much makeup and garish com-

binations. Even in a mild state of elation, the elated patient needs some supervision in this area.

3. Protection: He needs protection mainly from himself. He may give away all of his possessions. In an expansive mood, he may deed his property to someone else in a letter. He needs room to move around in, furnishings that don't overstimulate him.

4. Seclusion: Sometimes elated patients can be taught to monitor their own mounting hyperactivity and voluntarily go to a "quiet room" to reduce external stimuli. If a patient becomes more disturbed during seclusion he should be taken out immediately - if there are changes such as regression or quietness, he may be responding favorably to seclusion. Some clinicians see these changes as a breakthrough in the patient's psychosis, a "regression in the service of the ego", indicating that he's getting in touch with improved rationalizations and issues critical to him.

5. Recreation: He needs no encouragement to mingle with others, sometimes needs help to separate and walk alone. His short attention span and restless energy cannot deal with long-term or complicated projects. Needs tasks that are simple and quickly done. He enjoys writing and drawing and either activity is excellent therapy as well as rewarding recreation. In more aggressive moments, tearing and pounding also help him. He's rarely up to team sports while acutely elated and does better working at individual games or projects.

The elated patient is a human being first, and a patient second, just like every patient. The nurse's basic task with an elated patient is to maintain a calming, supportive, and structured environment in which he can decrease his tempo and develop some degree of control of his behavior. He needs protection from himself and his overactivity, physical care when his elation threatens his well-being (lack of food, lack of sleep), and calm reassurance that he is acceptable and can improve. His activities are planned to give him acceptable ways to expand his energy that are simple, quickly done and offer a means of expression, activities that help him function alone.

REVIEW QUESTIONS

1. How do elation and depression differ in psychodynamics?
2. What is the greatest danger to the patient while in an active elated period?
3. How are limits set?
4. What can be done with a patient who manipulates?
5. Why is physical care important for the elated patient?
6. What activities can be prescribed to help an elated patient?
7. How can seclusion be used therapeutically?

SUGGESTED REFERENCES

1. Almeida, E.M. and Chapman, A.H.: The Interpersonal Basis of Psychiatric Nursing, G.P. Putnam & Sons, New York, 1972

2. Arietti, S.: Manic-depressive psychosis, American Handbook of Psychiatry, Basic Books, Inc., New York, Vol. I, pp. 419-454, 1959

3. Brown, M.M. and Fowler, G.: Psychodynamic Nursing, W.B. Saunders, Philadelphia, 1971

4. Carigan, T.: Self-motivation and self-control in operant conditioning, Perspectives Psychi Care XII, 1974

5. Fitzgerald, R.G. and Long, I.: Seclusion in the treatment and management of severely disturbed manic and depressed patients, Perspectives Psychi Nursing XI:59-64, June, 1973

6. Kochansky, G.E.: Risk taking and hedonic mood stimulation in suicide attempters, J Abnormal Psychol LXXXI:80-86, Feb., 1973

7. Levitan, H.L.: Dreams preceding hypomania, International J Psychoanalytic Psychother I:50-61, May, 1972

8. Lenny, R.: Acting-out behavior of psychiatric nurses, Perspectives Psychi Care IV:10-14, 1966

9. Ujhely, G.B.: On being possessed by the devil, Perspectives Psychi Care X:202-209, Dec., 1972

10. Williams, D.H.: Sleep and disease, Am J Nursing LXXI:2321-2324, Dec., 1971

CHAPTER 8

THE WITHDRAWN PATIENT

Withdrawal is a behavior common to many psychiatric conditions from neurosis to organic disorders to depression. It is a component of almost any schizophrenic process.

Schizophrenic withdrawal is a form of breaking-off of contact with outer reality, and is one of the symptomatic behaviors in schizophrenia. Another symptom is restitution - restructuring a substitute world for the denied reality.

An elated or depressed patient may be absorbed in his own problems but still seems to maintain contact. The schizophrenic has a greater loss of contact and shows little or no interest in the world around him. In schizophrenia, the loss of the ego's adaptive capacity to neutralize aggression is defended against by withdrawal, projection and regression. The mechanism referred to as "splitting" separates the representations of self and objects, separating the two currents of strong feelings to reduce anxiety. Many of his symptoms express his denial; some of them express restitutive fantasies (hallucinations, delusions) in an effort to regain reality.

OVERT BEHAVIOR

1. Breaking-off symptoms:
   a. His speech may be unintelligible because he doesn't care whether he's understood or not. Having no interest in communicating, he talks in personal terms from within his fantasies rather than using speech to establish a relationship.
   b. His mood or affect is flat and he doesn't respond to the external world. May be very emotional about his delusions and fantasies without reacting to people or situations around him.
   c. He's inconsistent and disintegrated. His thinking, his feeling, and his behavior do not function harmoniously. Incongruity between ideas and affect, inability to stay with one idea for long. May be excited one moment and stuporous the next.
   d. He's uninhibited, doesn't care what anybody thinks and acts out impulsively. He no longer perceives the world as it is, nor deals with it as it is. He may use obscene language, masturbate in public, urinate on the walls, be openly hostile or shout and scream.
2. Restitutional symptoms:
   a. Delusions. False beliefs not changeable by appeal to reason. May have delusions of grandeur (greatness) and insist on being Christ, delusions of omnipotence (power) and fear that he can destroy the world by moving a finger, or delusions of persecution and think people are after him.
   b. Hallucinations. Sensory perceptions without external stimulus. May hear voices, smell odors, or feel something on his skin, see or taste things which are not there.

86

These symptoms are never meaningless. The patient tries to accomplish something with his symptoms but doesn't succeed. The anger and anxiety often displayed with restitutional behavior would suggest that the delusions or hallucinations are not working.

In catatonia, the acute, suddenly occurring form of withdrawal, the underlying dynamics are exaggerated. The patient is completely helpless, assuming stances and postures (waxy flexibilities) and automatically doing as directed (automatism) in a robot-unhuman-like fashion. Repeating words (ecolalia) and actions of others (ecopraxia), the picture of total dependency on external control is sharply contrasted with the unpredictable frenzy of the excitement stage during which the intensely repressed anger and hostility burst forth in rage and violence. It is the inadequacy of the withdrawal defense and the uncontrolled expression of anger that gives catatonia the best prognosis of the schizophrenia subtypes.

PSYCHODYNAMICS

There are many approaches to the problem of schizophrenic etiology. Familial tendencies, physiological differences, and family relationships are only some of the factors studied. Research in genetics (Kaplan), family relationships (Despert) and, more recently, orthomolecular therapy with vitamins (Hawkins, Ross) has left the question of schizophrenic etiology still unanswered.

In terms of the ego, the schizophrenic has a weak ego which is unable to function as mediator between self and external reality. As the reality becomes more threatening, he cuts it off, regressing to a previous developmental stage. As the regression increases, the ego and the superego are further weakened and the id is free to break through. The feelings are threatening and so are isolated from the ideas or actions and are repressed.

In Piagetian developmental theory, the schizophrenic can't form concepts or think abstractly. His thinking is concrete, animistic (endowing inanimate objects with purpose and power) and completely egocentric. Such an interruption in cognitive development leaves the individual with an inability to think on an adult level although not necessarily lacking in intelligence. He has problems assimilating new information into present structures, leaving the structure unable to function adequately.

Instead of just one causative factor, schizophrenia probably results from a combination of many factors: individual adaptive patterns, ego strength, family relationships, experiences, biological abnormalities and the cognitive development.

NURSING INTERVENTIONS

Main focus is to bring him back to reality:

1. Communication:
   a. Establish a positive relationship (without it little is accomplished).

    b. Approach him at his present level of functioning.
    c. Broaden his contacts to include other people.
    d. Emphasize everday present-oriented nonthreatening topics
       until a closer relationship is established.
    e. Reflect his feelings, and try to rebuild his self-esteem.
    f. Accept testing-out behaviors such as withdrawal, negativism,
       and hostility.
2. Stress reality: Point out inappropriate behavior, stay out of his
   hallucinations, observe for precipitating factors and intervene
   before hallucination occurs. Try to distract him from delusions
   with other things.

The psychodynamics of hallucinations, a primary symptom in the
diagnosis of schizophrenia, are very complex. Hallucinations have
three fundamental characteristics:

1. The created perception.
2. The projection of the created perception into the real world.
3. The inability of the hallucinating person to discern that it is a
   created perception (Arieti).

Hallucinations usually begin in an anxious, lonely person under stress.
The content of hallucinations replaces relationships the person
once had with others. Having no "helping" person around, he autistically invents auditory hallucinations.

Peplau has identified seven sequential phases in the development of
auditory hallucinations.

Phase I - Recall of a helping person relieves the person's anxiety.

Phase II - In a subsequent anxiety situation, the person repeats the re-
lief-giving behavior and relief is felt and a ritual is established.
This private frame of reference is increasingly used; the content of
the hallucinations are from past and present materials.

Phase III - The person begins to doubt his ability to interact with his
invented friend; because of the relief he has experienced, he sets
aside more time for hallucinatory experiences and less time with
real people. He withdraws and this causes a loss of first, compe-
tency in interacting with real people, and second, the ability to maintain the focus of his attention.

Phase IV - Further reduction of focal attention causing others to
notice the hallucinatory behavior. This evokes criticism leading to
more anxiety and thus more hallucinating which alleviates this
anxiety.

Phase V - Derogatory elements in the self-system are incorporated
into the invented figure. Voices are now derogatory instead of supportive. The relief behavior (hallucinations) no longer relieves
anxiety.

Phase VI - Derogatory - "voices" now become unacceptable "not me".
They are accusatory; he has "disowned them". Other

problems: loss of focal awareness; increased withdrawal; increased anxiety. Abstract voice (or voices) are now concrete, he feels they control him and he isn't responsible for his own behavior (thus he suffers from his own fragmented recollections).

Phase VII - Compromising with voices to appease them. Voices threaten, terrorize him. If he discovers they lie to him, he may be able to distrust them, combat them, and with therapy, dismiss them.

The following approach to patients who are hallucinating has been suggested:

1. Have the patient name the fact of being anxious and connect behavior with it. This is necessary in order to have any control over the hallucinating process.
2. Acquire a relationship with the patient. Talk about other events, not just the hallucinations.
3. Do not afford the voices any status, respecting that this is the patient's experience. Refer to the voices as "so-called voices".
4. The patient himself must dismiss the voices. A time of terror and high anxiety may follow a patient's dismissal of voices.
5. When the time approaches for the dismissal of the voices, the nurse makes sure that other staff members become interested in the patient and provide temporary replacement for the invented figures (Peplau).

Delusions, false beliefs and interpretations and exaggerations of facts which are the unrecognized expression of repressed or dissociated materials (Fromm Reichman, p. 176). Delusions are attempts to alter reality which is unacceptable due to a strong unconscious need. Three defenses are prominent and develop sequentially:

1. A segment of reality is denied.
2. Feelings and thoughts are projected to the environment and viewed as coming from outside.
3. This interpretation of reality is rationalized to self and others (Freud).

Delusions develop because something definite exists on which scattered attention can be focused and they usually have some base in reality. Thus, the patient suffers from his own distorted recollections.

The nursing approach develops from the decoding of the delusion. The sequential steps are:

1. Careful alert listening to the delusion to untangle the historical and dynamic roots of the delusion.
2. Identify elements of reality, noting the relationship of the delusional contents to the patient's behavior.
3. Hypothesize the symbolically expressed need(s) that are being met by the delusion. If there is a delusional system, examine it to find organizing elements.
4. Ignore the delusional system and have others on staff do the same.

5. Set limit that patient is not to discuss the delusional material saying, "You do not benefit from this topic discussion" or some such comment.
6. Structure situation so patient cannot get into delusional discussions (activities, brief encounters).
7. Intervene by working on the problem (need) the delusion represents, not the delusion itself.
8. Evaluation of hypothesis by patient's decreased need to use delusion (Dixson).

Needs most commonly expressed through the symbolic delusion (or hallucinations, which are dynamically related) are needs for self-esteem (as in psychotically depressed), hostility (as in paranoid and sexual expression), and dependency and trust (as in paranoid schizophrenia).

Many withdrawn patients retreat from verbal communications and are labeled "mute" or "noncommunicative". The sounds of silence may have many causes. In addition to the usual explanations of negativism and stubborness, he may be nonverbal because:

1. By not hearing verbalizations of his thoughts, it may be easier for the patient to deny they exist.
2. He may be fearful of the reactions of others to what he says.
3. He may have limitations in formulating his reactions since he didn't develop the ability to verbalize strong feelings.
4. He may be using resistance, punishing others by withholding self-revelations.
5. By withholding information he may be using a means of control, both of himself and of others.
6. He may have irrational ideas as to the magical power of his thoughts, and verbalizations may be synonomous with actions to him.
7. He may have a limited capacity for intimacy and social inertia.
8. He may have a lack of differentiation between himself and the outside world and attribute to others "mind-reading" abilities.
9. He may have pathological, exaggerated notions of the complications and dangers of an interpersonal relationship.
10. He may fear dependency on the therapist, a re-enactment of parental or an addition to the externally controlling forces that already impinge on his weak ego.
11. Without language, the task of the potential receiver is so great he won't bother (unless he has an extreme need to control or incorporate others). Aware of the repelling nature of his silent defense, the patient thus perceives anyone attempting intervention as having a one-sided relatedness problem. By stereotyping reaction of others, he sees the sender as dangerous and retreats more (Rouslin).

The silent treatment is often an affective approach to the silent patient, i.e., using silence to intervene in silence. By sharing the patients' silence, the nurse:

1. Exerts no pressure (control) on the patient to talk. By her
   silent presence, she shows she is willing to wait and provide the
   time needed.
2. Her "comfortable" sharing of his silent stance conveys that it is
   okay to be silent, that silent behavior is not objectionable, bad,
   or "sick".
3. By her silent, calm presence, she indicates she will wait for the
   patient to communicate and knows he has the ability. Thus, she
   is appealing to the healthy part of his ego that wants to talk.
4. By not probing, interrogating, or carrying on a one-sided dialogue, the patient is reassured of the nurse's motives. If asked
   to talk, the patient feels he must obey the therapist, precipitating
   transferences which put the patient back in the infantile, dependent role which originally overwhelmed him. This results in more
   distancing, guilt, and a retrenched silence.
5. By not permitting transference, the patient is not required to obey
   therapist and he is encouraged to assume responsibility for his
   own actions (talking).
6. By accepting the silence comfortably, the nurse lessens the anxiety and guilt the patient may be experiencing by not talking. The
   lessening of tension may open up the dialogue and he may begin
   to talk.

3. Physical Care:
   a. May retain feces and urine; needs to be observed closely, re-
      conditioned, encouraged to exercise.
   b. Has difficulty with food and fluids, may not be interested, un-
      able to decide what to do first, afraid to eat, or physically
      unable to eat. May have to be fed.
   c. Neglects his personal appearance and needs help in making
      decisions. Has to have instructions offered in concrete
      terms step-by-step.
   d. May have difficulty sleeping - or difficulty staying awake.
      Needs to know why he can't sleep before effective help can be
      given.
4. Protection: He needs to be protected from himself and others
   need to be protected from him. He may attack others or try to
   destroy himself while hallucinating or delusional.
5. Recreation: Needs simple concrete tasks in which he is actively
   involved. Metal work and modeling clay are effective beginning
   tasks using his sense of touch and giving him a chance to be
   creative.

Group activities help him adjust to the real world once he has made
some contact with a few individuals. Dancing, noncompetitive ath-
letics, outings - all are excellent therapy.

It is most important that the nurse be interested in the patient, recognize her own feelings, and be honest, accepting, and supportive
in behavior. The nurse's basic task with a withdrawn patient is to
help the patient improve his contact with reality by assisting him in
decreasing the interpersonal gulf existing between him and others.
He needs protection from himself (especially when hallucinating or
delusional), physical care when his withdrawal affects his health
(bowel and bladder problems, inability to eat or sleep, inappropri-

ate clothing), and empathic reassurance of his self-worth. His activities are planned to give him simple, concrete (yet creative) tasks and to help him function within a group (picnics, ward meetings, games).

REVIEW QUESTIONS

1. What is restitution?
2. What are some of the signs of a "flat affect"?
3. What is the etiology of schizophrenia?
4. How can Piaget's developmental theory explain schizophrenia?
5. What is the first priority in nursing the schizophrenic patient?
6. How do hallucinations and delusions differ?
7. How can restitutional symptoms be altered?

SUGGESTED REFERENCES

1. Anderson, N.: Suicide in schizophrenia, Perspectives Psychi Care XI:406-413, 1973

2. Arnold, H.: Four A's: Guide to one-to-one relationships, Am J Nursing, pp. 941-943, June, 1976

3. Arieti, S.: Interpretation of Schizophrenia, Basic Books, Inc., New York, 1955

4. Arieti, S.: The Intra-Psychic Self, Basic Books, Inc., New York, 1967

5. Astendoff, M.: Dane's schizophrenia: Possible causes, probable cause, Am J Nursing, pp. 947-948, June, 1976

6. Cloud, E.D.: The plateau, Perspectives Psychi Care X:112-121, 1972

7. Field, W. and Ruelke, W.: Hallucinations and how to deal with them, Am J Nursing, pp. 638-640, April, 1973

8. Grand, S., et al.: A study of the representation of objects in schizophrenia, J Am Psychoanalytic Assoc XXI:379-393, 1973

9. Goodwin, D.W., et al.: Clinical significance of hallucinations in psychiatric disorders, Arch Gen Psychi XXIV:76-80, 1971

10. Hawkins, D. and Pauling, L., Ed.: Orthomolecular Psychiatry, W.H. Freeman & Co., San Francisco, 1973

11. Jackson, D.: The Etiology of Schizophrenia, Basic Books, Inc., New York, 1960

12. Kaplan, A., Ed.: Genetic Factors in Schizophrenia, Charles C. Thomas, Springfield, Ill., 1972

13. Laing, R.D.: The Divided Self, Penguin Books, Maryland, 1965

14. Lichtenberg, J.D. and Stap, J.W.: Notes on the concept of splitting and the defense mechanism of splitting of representations, J Am Psychoanalytical Assoc XXI:772-789, 1972

15. Lowe, G.R.: The phenomenology of hallucinations as an aid to differential diagnosis, Br J Psychi, pp. 621-633, Dec., 1973

16. Masher, L.R., et al.: Identical twins discordant for schizophrenia, Arch Gen Psychi XXIV:422-430, 1971

17. Mickens: The influence of the therapist on resistive silences, Perspectives Psychi Care I:161-166, 1971

18. Robinson, G.: Reaching to be free, Am J Nursing, pp. 944-947, 1976

19. Ross, H.M.: Orthomolecular psychiatry, vitamin pills for schizophrenia, Psychol Today VII:82-87, April, 1974

20. Searles, H.F.: Intensive psychotherapy of chronic schizophrenia, International J Psychoanalytic Psychother I:30-51, May, 1972

21. Sechehaye, M.A.: Symbolic Realization, International Universities Press, Inc., New York, 1951

22. Stevens, J.R.: An anatomy of schizophrenia, Arch Gen Psychi XXIX:177-189, 1973

23. Tudor, G.: A sociopsychiatric nursing approach to intervention in a problem of mutual withdrawal on a mental hospital ward, (Reprint), Perspectives Psychi Care VIII:11-48, 1970

24. Ujhley, G.: Nursing intervention with the acutely ill psychiatric patient, Nursing Forum VIII:311-326, 1969

25. Wright: A symbolic tree: Loneliness is the roots; delusions are the leaves, J Psychi Nursing Mental Health Sci, XIII:30-35 May-June, 1975

26. Yarden, P.E. and Discipio, W.J.: Abnormal movements and prognosis in schizophrenia, Am J Psychi CXXVIII:317-323, 1971

CHAPTER 9

THE SUSPICIOUS PATIENT

The suspicious person is called "paranoid" and may be viewed with some distaste by others. Paranoid, or suspicious tendencies are shared by the senile, the alcoholic, the brain-damaged, and the schizophrenic. In a recent study (Lowe), paranoid patients are differentiated from schizophrenic manic-depressive and brain-damaged individuals on the basis of their hallucinations. Five variables accounted for 66-78 percent of the differences between groups and excluded 69-90 percent of possible wrong diagnoses.

Paranoid hallucinations differed in number (fewer), in duration (almost incessant) and modality (auditory), in content (concerned others in negative or threatening situations), in overt behavior (physical activity) and in whether the experience was thought to be shared (thought others knew about and shared in the hallucination).

The paranoid personality is a sensitive personality. The individual's attitude towards others is one of suspicion. The "paranoid position" is a feeling of constant persecution.

Paranoia develops on a continuum from suspicion to ideas of reference (fixed false ideas that all conversation, laughter, etc. refer to him) to delusions of persecution to delusions of grandeur. Projection of his suspicions upon others and thinking they are going to harm or kill him makes the paranoid person the most dangerous of all patients. He develops a paranoid community or the fixed focus on specific persons as the source of danger. The community is an imaginary organization but includes real people, misidentified people and imaginary people. "They" are all conspirators against the paranoid individual. Real happenings and trivial incidents are all given great significance to support the idea of a community conspiracy. As the community becomes larger, the individual becomes less able to control it. If he acts out his suspicions in aggressive acts against his "enemies", the almost inevitable counter-aggression reaffirms his delusional expectation of attack.

The paranoid personality is tense, insecure, rigid, secretive and seclusive. He finds people untrustworthy and has great difficulty in assuming the role of another person and trying to view things from a different perspective. He is unduly concerned with other people's opinion of him and he is incompetent in cooperative or complimentary relationships. A dominant delusional individual can induce a parallel delusion in a dependent person. When the partners in this "folie a deux" are separated, the dependent one recovers quickly, the dominant one does not.

In Freudian terms, the paranoid person's use of denial and projection fails to protect his ego against repressed homosexual wishes and fears of castration. In Sullivanian terms, there is parataxic distortion and danger from even his significant others. In Eriksonian terms, basic trust has never developed but basic mistrust has become a driving force. In Piagetian terms, extreme egocentrism prevents seeing another's point of view and excessive centering distorts the world.

Whether or not a paranoid idea is considered psychotic, neurotic, or normal, depends upon how many people believe it. Hitler blamed the troubles of Germany on non-Aryans and was considered a leader. Almost every president in modern times considered the press "unfriendly and out-to-get him" and has been called paranoid. It's a matter of degree and emphasis.

OVERT BEHAVIOR

1. Interprets interpersonal relationships in terms of being persecuted. Reacts excessively to rebuff, becomes suspicious and rejected again.
2. May have only one area of fixed delusion - functions well until paranoid concept is activated.
3. Self-accusatory auditory hallucinations if functional; life endangering visual hallucinations, if organic.
4. Delusions of superiority, of persecution.
5. Acts upon delusions and hallucinations with sarcasm, sneering, aggression, and violence.

PSYCHODYNAMICS

Projection, narcissism and self-absorption blur the ego boundaries or the distinctions between the self and external reality. The individual has within him much unacknowledged and poorly integrated violence and guilt. He also has poor interpersonal relationships.

He regresses to an archaic state in which he "incorporates" and then "projects" his bad conscience into the external world as a persecutor. The superego, as an introjected object of the same sex when projected leads to fears and an overdefense against homosexuality, although he's not necessarily homosexual.

Fears of aggression and retaliation interfere with the normal resolution of his Oedipal conflict. He doesn't have a clear picture of himself as male or female, doesn't feel a sense of control of himself or his impulses.

He develops paranoid ideas in an attempt to organize his frightening feelings into some sort of logical system in order to make some sense out of them.

NURSING INTERVENTIONS

1. Communication:
   a. Use simple clear language and avoid physical contact so that he won't misinterpret words, actions, or meanings.
   b. Avoid power struggles. Accept his superior, sarcastic behavior calmly.
   c. Give support by being self-assured and nonpunitive.

    d. Avoid using logic and trying to reason with him.

    e. Acknowledge his fears, and direct his attention to other activities.

2. <u>Physical Needs</u>:

    a. Diet - may refuse to eat for fear of being poisoned. Let him fix own meals, eat out of original containers, or eat with him.

    b. Sleep - may be afraid to sleep, unable to sleep with others.

    c. Appearance - can probably take care of his own needs, may resent any attempts of the nurse to help.

3. <u>Protection</u>: Always a threat to others and to himself. Protect him during hallucinations, and observe him closely at all times.

4. <u>Recreation</u>: Noncompetitive solitary tasks that require some degree of concentration. Don't expect him to compete with others or even to cooperate with them. Jigsaw puzzles, crosswords, ceramics are all good therapy, because they require close concentration and leave less time for concentrating on delusions. They are all solitary, noncompetitive activities which require no physical contact yet utilize small and large muscles as well as cognitive functions.

Paranoid symptoms are also observable in old age and in involutional melancholia. The symptoms are far more prevalent than the disease.

The nurse's basic task with a paranoid patient is to lessen his feelings of guilt and rejection and to help him into closer contact with reality. He needs to be protected during hallucinations and prevented from harming others. Although he is usually able to care for himself physically, intervention may be necessary if he cannot sleep or is afraid to eat. He responds to noncompetitive, solitary activities which use his muscles and his mind and require close concentration.

REVIEW QUESTIONS

1. What can be done for the suspicious patient who won't eat?
2. How do his delusions affect his behavior?
3. What would constitute a self-accusatory auditory hallucination?
4. Is there any relationship between paranoid delusions and homosexuality?
5. What are the important things to remember in planning recreational activities for the suspicious patient?
6. Why are fewer people being diagnosed as paranoid today?
7. Why are paranoids so alert to their environment?

SUGGESTED REFERENCES

1. Artiss, K.L. and Bullard, D.M.: Paranoid thinking in everyday life, <u>Arch Gen Psychi</u>, pp. 95-112, 1966

2. Brown, M.M. and Fowler, G.: <u>Psychodynamic Nursing</u>, W.B. Saunders, Philadelphia, 1971

3. Cameron, N.: Paranoid conditions and paranoia, <u>American Handbook of Psychiatry</u>, Basic Books, Inc., New York, 3rd Ed., Arieti, S., Ed., pp. 676-699, 1974

4. Chrzanowski, J.: Cultural and pathological manifestations of paranoias, Discussions (Ujhely), Perspectives Psychi Care IV: 43-49, 1965

5. Ingraham, M.: Comprehensive study of a psychiatric patient (paranoid), Perspectives Psychi Care II:22-26, 1964

6. Izard, C.E.: Paranoid schizophrenics and normal subject perception of photographs of human faces, J Consulting Psychol XXIII:119-124, 1959

7. Mellow, J.: Experiential order of nursing therapy in acute schizophrenia, Perspectives Psychi Care VI:249-260, 1968

8. Mereness, D.: Essentials of Psychiatric Nursing, C.V. Mosby, St. Louis, 1970

9. Noyes, A., et al.: Psychiatric Nursing, The Macmillan Co., New York, 1964

10. Pinderhughes, C.A.: Managing paranoid violent relationships, Perspectives on Violence, Usdin, G., Ed., Brunner-Mazel, New York, 1972

11. Schatzman, M.: Paranoia or persecution: The case of Schreber, International J Psychi X:53-78, Sept., 1972

12. Stankiewicz: Guides to nursing intervention in the projective patterns of suspicious patients, Perspectives Psychi Care II:39-45, 1964

13. Varables, P. and O'Connor, N.: A short scale for rating paranoid schizophrenia, Mental Sci LV:815-818, 1959

CHAPTER 10

THE ANTISOCIAL PATIENT

Usually only the "sociopath" is called antisocial, but child and substance abusers also fit into this category. The sociopath's problems with society are usually legal; the drug addict's are legal and medical; the alcoholic's are now primarily medical; the child abuser's are legal but his victim's are medical.

There seems little difference to society if, instead of being robbed or murdered by a sociopath, the stealing is done by a drug addict or the killing by a drunken driver or a child abuser.

Each one shows a remarkable lack of concern for other people. There are differences in the behavior and care and similarities in the dynamics of antisocial patients.

Research (Berzin's) shows that addicts (drugs or alcohol) can be categorized into two groups: (1) inadequate, hypersensitive, alienated, confused, deviant, more psychiatric than sociopathic and treatable; and (2) adjusted, outgoing, poised, optimistic deviant sociopaths, for whom treatment is a game and drugs or alcohol are ego syntonic.

OVERT BEHAVIOR

1. The sociopath. Charming and intelligent at first, on closer observation he is superficial, inconsistent, untruthful, performs the same acts repeatedly, not learning from experience, doesn't express affection. He states what is right or wrong, legal or illegal, but his actions differ. Actions appear unplanned; he follows whichever course seems easiest at the moment. He manipulates others, doesn't form close or lasting relationships and may be a sexual deviant. Callous, emotionally immature, he shows poor judgment, but rationalizes his behavior so that others find him reasonable. He remains personable and charming to others, communicating freely, manipulating and causing considerable friction.
2. Drug addict. Emotionally immature, dependent, passive, self-destructive. Inarticulate, limited conversation, may be apathetic or hyperactive. Unimaginative, easily frustrated, and has a short attention span. Often untruthful and insincere. May be elated or depressed while on drugs and have weight loss, elevated temperature, constipation or diarrhea. Withdrawal symptoms: anxiety, muscular twitching and tremors, sneezing, yawning, sweating, "watery eyes", "goose flesh", vomiting, fever, abdominal cramps, dehydration and (with drugs such as barbiturates) convulsions.
3. Alcoholic. Usually talks easily with others, resents authority, has a low frustration tolerance, is dependent, domineering, and selfish in his demands. Untruthful and insincere, professes

shame and promises never to drink again. May be anxious or depressed, have insomnia, fine tremors, thirst, perspiration, slurred speech, chronic liver or brain damage, and delirium tremens (DT's). Symptoms of DT's: extreme agitation, frenzied activity, fear, disorientation, poor coordination, coarse tremors, thirst, sweating, and hallucination.

4. The child abuser. Likable but immature. He is impatient, has poor impulse control, low frustration tolerance. He is self-centered and narcissistic but with a poor self-concept. He will lie about the child's condition and take him to a different doctor or hospital each time. He often blames other children in the family or in the neighborhood for the injuries.

PSYCHODYNAMICS

"Character" is a person's typical individual pattern of adaptation, his habitual way of dealing with the world. Character is a product of the ego, the integrating force which determines how anyone will deal with internal conflicts and external problems. The ego begins developing early in life; character develops as the early developmental stages are successfully negotiated.

If a child's dependency needs can be satisfied by his parent figures while he is also learning to give as well as take, to adapt his own needs to the needs of others; if he is allowed to be aggressive yet taught the limitations of social living; then his character development is likely to proceed smoothly.

Neurotic, psychotic, antisocial and deviant individuals are all involved with problems that should have been resolved long before. They are concerned with such basic and infantile things as wanting to be dependent or aggressive.

The ego mediates between id and superego. In the elated patient, the ego capitulates to the id; in the depressed the ego capitulates to the superego. In the antisocial types the ego capitulates to both, and the battle is between id and superego.

The elated individual acts out his id impulses and is not punished. The depressed individual is punished without having acted out his id impulses. The antisocial individual acts out, is punished, acts out, is punished - repeatedly.

Not having learned to give as well as take, the antisocial individual is a taker and views others as being there to satisfy his needs. Without a strong ego function he can develop a close relationship with no one. He remains narcissistic and orally-oriented and views reality in an inappropriate egocentric manner.

He views himself unrealistically and expects much more than he can satisfy. When he cannot live up to his expectation of himself, the anxiety and guilt become intolerable. He regresses to the infantile behavior that was once rewarded and substitutes his oral need satisfaction for a mature love relationship.

The sociopath sometimes turns to alcohol or drugs to satisfy his oral needs but more commonly he satisfies them with conversation or sex. The drug addict, of course, satisfies his oral needs with drugs, the alcoholic with alcohol and the child abuser with verbal abuse and biting. The child abuser, not satisfied with his sex role projects his dissatisfaction upon the child.

By being helpless, sick, unable to cope with society and always in trouble, they can again assume dependent roles in their families or have social agencies and law enforcers take the responsibility for controlling their impulses.

Each one can deny reality and be the superior and accomplished individual he feels himself to be - in fantasy, or in sexual acting-out.

Like the phobic individual who invests his anxiety in external objects that can be avoided, the antisocial individual invests his in external objects that can be incorporated or destroyed. The phobic individual avoids his anxiety, the antisocial type tries to swallow his - orally or sexually and the child abuser projects his upon another human being.

Often a product of dysfunctional parenting, the child abuser was himself abused and identified with the aggressor. A poor self-image from his parents plus parental abuse leads to suspicion of authority. He acts out in response to ambivalent emotions and confusion in parental and child roles. He expects more from the child than the child can provide and, in anger and frustration, abuses - and often kills - the child. Child abuse is one of the leading causes of death in children and has increased tenfold in the last 10 years.

The phobic punishes himself, the antisocial individual needs external gratification and external punishment. He runs afoul of society repeatedly and consistently. Unable to control either his impulses or his guilt, he seeks someone else who can control and punish him. Then he frustrates and "beats" the one who would help him by refusing to change and leaving the therapists to face failure.

In recent years, the concept of "borderline" personalities has gained wide usage in the literature. In borderline psychopathology, the "splitting" mechanism occurs during the infantile period as in psychoses; however, the feelings "split" are absorbed by the forming ego to become a character trait. In the psychotic, the split feelings are repressed and precursors to anxiety and guilt; in the borderline patient they evolve to a nonthreatening, character trait. Borderline character disorders are a response to a series of psychically traumatic events rather than the specific events frequently seen in the psychoses or neuroses.

NURSING INTERVENTIONS

1. Sociopath. This individual will communicate easily and enter into a relationship quickly. He will trust no one and manipulate everyone. Close observation is needed to identify his behavior. He needs a consistency and firmness from the nurse and variety of treatments and activities. Physical care is almost never

necessary. Intelligent and appealing, he is easily bored and begins dominating and using others. Other patients need to be protected from him; he will often obtain dangerous objects such as
matches, drugs, knives, or alcohol for them. He manipulates
with tears, lies, and threats and uses staff against staff, staff
against family, family against staff, to get what he wants. All
the staff involved with the patient need to exchange information
to minimize his attempts to play one against the other. The
nurse needs to be calm, quiet, firm and consistent, never expecting him to be more or better than he is. Long discussions
lead to concessions or tantrums, which in turn lead to further
manipulation, so explanations are more effective when brief and
clear. If he is viewed as a patient with a certain type of pathology, the nurse will be less apt to expect behaviors of which he
is incapable; she will accept him as he is and not be angry or
hurt when he uses and threatens her.

2. Drug addict.
   a. Detoxification. Five to seven days, longer for females than
      for males. Sleep patterns during detoxification differ for
      males (at night) and females (day). Focus on friendly, unin-
      volved supportive therapy since high anxiety may cause him
      to leave treatment center. Two approaches are recom-
      mended: frequent, brief one-to-one supportive encounters
      focusing on physical symptoms, and a medical regime to
      raise the blood sugar level. Nursing, not addiction therapy,
      should be the major focus to alleviate problems.
   b. Recovery Phase. Inarticulate and withdrawn, needs help in
      communicating. May have severe anxiety and depression.
      Since self-medication is frequently an effort to control ag-
      gressive impulses, acting out of aggressions can be antici-
      pated when the controlling drug effects have been withdrawn.

      The role of the nurse in therapy may differ in different areas.
      She may be able to actively enter into the process of changing
      the addict's behavior as a member of the psychiatric team,
      or she may merely care for his physical needs and have little
      part in his psychological care. No matter what the limita-
      tions of her role, the nurse can try to help him with his com-
      munication problems, help him broaden his interests with
      music, art, or vocational courses, maintain realistic goals
      for him so he doesn't become discouraged, and protect him
      from drugs that someone may bring in.

3. Alcoholic. May be in a chronic or acute state.
   a. Acute state. Mainly physical care, fluid and vitamin therapy,
      perhaps gavage. Keep his room well lighted and free of ex-
      traneous objects to help alleviate hallucinatory behavior.
      Help with food when tremors are too intense for him to use
      his hands. No lectures - his behavior has meaning and is the
      best he can manage at the moment. He needs support, firm-
      ness. He may deny his condition; the nurse needs to identify
      it and help him face it. Needs protection from himself - may
      jump out of the window in delirium, or drink his mouthwash
      when he can hold the bottle.

Patients who develop hallucinations while withdrawing from alcohol are usually those who have been confined to bed and restrained and/or sedated. The hallucinatory syndrome is similar to that of elderly patients whose environment has been changed. Neither need occur if the approach is a nonthreatening supportive atmosphere and frequent contacts with friends or peers for reality orientation.

b. Chronic state. No longer needs much physical care. Important for him to care for himself. Needs support and help in understanding his actions and encouragement to seek further therapy. Needs acceptance of himself as an individual but not as an alcoholic. Will try to manipulate, promise to change, but have alcohol brought in by someone else. Needs to have his behavior pointed out to him and needs help in facing himself. Needs protection from possible suicide attempts when he becomes depressed or frustrated.

4. Child abuser. Because of his problems with authority, it is difficult to establish a therapeutic relationship. The nurse needs to develop a therapeutic posture and act as a role model, gratify his dependency needs and provide good parent experiences. Teach him how to relate to others, how to make friends and model for him how to act. Teach him about normal child development so that he does not expect adult behavior from a six-month-old baby or four-year-old child.

Any antisocial individual has problems facing his behavior, seeing himself as he is. Always promising to do better, they live out a type of role reversal in their families with antisocial fathers or mothers playing the role of the dependent child.

The poorest prognosis for any kind of psychological treatment is in antisocial personalities.

Their masochism results in punishment-seeking behavior but these individuals are also sadistic enough to hurt others by their behavior. The hostility is so great they repeatedly make other people suffer, and repeatedly refuse to let others help them.

The nurse's basic task with an antisocial patient is to reinforce reality and to maintain control while protecting other patients from him, as well as protecting him from himself and others. Physical care is rarely needed except in either acute or withdrawal states. Activities that enhance his self-esteem and are expressive and creative but not too complicated are best.

REVIEW QUESTIONS

1. Does the sociopath know "right from wrong"?
2. How do substance and child abusers differ?
3. What sort of nursing care does an alcoholic require? A drug addict?
4. What are the dynamics of the antisocial personality?
5. Who suffers the most from antisocial behavior - the individual with the behavior, or society as a whole?
6. Why do people abuse children instead of substances?

SUGGESTED REFERENCES

1. Anthony, E.J. and Kreitman, N.: Murderous obsessions in mothers toward their children, Parenthood Its Psychology and Psychopathology, Anthony E.J. and Benedek, T., Eds., Little, Brown & Co., Inc., Boston, 1970

2. Berzins, J.I., et al.: Subgroups among opiate addicts: A typological investigation, J Abnormal Psychol LXXXIII:65-73, Feb., 1974

3. Brink, P.: Heroin addicts: Return of behavior during detoxification, J Psychi Nursing Mental Health Sci, pp. 12-18, April, 1972

4. Brody, E.: Borderline States: Character Disorder and Psychotic Manifestations - Some Conceptual Formulations, Psychiatry XXIII:75-80, Feb., 1960

5. Chafetz, M.E.: The prevention of alcoholism, International J Psychi IX:329-348, Aronson, J., Ed., Science House, 1970

6. Childress, G.: The role of the nurse with the drug abuser and addict, J Psychi Nursing VIII:21-26, March-April, 1970

7. Clef, V.: The hostility of parents to children: Some notes on infertility, child abuse and abortion, International J Psychotherapy, Feb., 1972

8. Copel, S.: Juvenile delinquency, Behavior Pathology of Childhood and Adolescence, Copel, S.J., Ed., Basic Books, Inc., New York, 1973

9. Gelles, R.J.: The social construction of child abuse, Am J Orthopsychi XLIII:363-371, April, 1975

10. Govoni, L.E. and Hayes, J.E.: Drugs and Nursing Implications, Appleton-Century-Crofts, New York, 1971

11. Helfer, R.E.: The Diagnostic Process and Treatment Programs, Child Abuse, U.S. Dept. of Health, Education and Welfare, DHEW, Pub. No. OHD, U.S. Printing Office, Washington, D.C., pp.69-75, 1975

12. Kempe, C., et al.: The battered child syndrome, J Am Med Assoc, pp. 17-24, July, 1962

13. Meninger, K.: Man Against Himself, Harcourt, Brace & World, Inc., New York, 1938

14. Mitchell, C.E.: Assessment of alcohol abuse, Nursing Outlook XXIV:511-515, Aug., 1976

15. Kernberg, O.F.: Prognostic considerations regarding borderline personality organization, J Am Psychoanalytic Assoc XIX: 595-635, 1971

16. Mack, J.E.: Borderline states, Psychiatric Seminars in Psychiatry, Greenblatt, M., Ed., Grune & Stratton, New York, 1975

17. Mueller, J.F.: Treatment for the alcoholic: Cursing or nursing? Am J Nursing LXXIV:245-247, Feb., 1974

18. Pillari, G. and Narus, J.: Physical Effects of Heroin Addiction LXXIII:2105-2108, Dec., 1973

19. Poplar, J.: Characteristics of nurse addicts, Am J Nursing LXIX:117-119, Jan., 1969

20. Rodewald, R.: Speed kills: The adolescent methedrine addict, Perspectives Psychi Care VIII:160-168, April, 1970

21. Saul, L.J.: Dynamics of cigarette addiction, International J Psychoanalytic Psychother I:24-29, May, 1972

22. Spinettia, J.J., et al.: The child abusing parent: A psychological review, Psychological Bull LXXVII:296-304, April, 1972

23. Steiner, C.: Games Alcoholics Play, Grove Press, Inc., New York, 1971

24. Wheat, P.: By Sanction of the Victim, Major Books, Chatsworth, Calif., 1976

25. Wurmiser, L.: Drug abuse: Nemesis of psychiatry, International J Psychi X:94-107, Dec., 1972

CHAPTER 11

THE DEVIANT PATIENT

Sexual deviation prior to the twentieth century was a punishable offense, sometimes punishable by death. Even today such deviation is defined as a socially condemned variation of "normal" sexual conduct.

Great changes have occurred in the degree of social acceptance of deviation during the late sixties and early seventies. Laws reflect the change from ostracism to the acceptance of behavior between adults as being a private matter.

OVERT BEHAVIOR

There are many ways to achieve sexual gratification:

1. Exhibitionism - exposing genitals in public.
2. Voyeurism - watching others in erotic acts.
3. Fetishism - manipulating external objects.
4. Masturbation - manipulating own genitals.
5. Masochism - receiving pain from another.
6. Sadism - inflicting pain upon another.
7. Rape - forcing another to have intercourse.
8. Pedophilia - having sexual activity with a child.
9. Incest - having intercourse with blood relations (especially mother and son, father and daughter).
10. Necrophilia - having intercourse with the dead.
11. Transvestism - wearing clothes of the opposite sex.
12. Homosexuality - having sexual relationships with the same sex.

Rapists, child molesters or other deviates are most often seen in jail or in the community. The homosexual is the sex deviate most often seen in psychiatric nursing although not usually because of the homosexuality.

Male homosexuals and female homosexuals differ in their behavior, the male behavior having been studied more extensively. Males enter into more frequent and shorter relationships, are youth-oriented, and are more often anal in practices. Females have fewer and longer lasting relationships, are not youth-oriented, and are more oral in practices.

Either male or female may be cold, self-centered, sarcastic and hostile. They display behaviors characteristic of the earliest oral and anal stages of development, are impatient, sulky, dependent yet rebellious, and try to blame others for their own mistakes. Although considered as deviating from societal norms, they are conformists within their own groups, egocentric and have their own vocabulary of "code" words with which to identify contacts.

Homosexuals may be seductive toward staff or other patients and latent homosexuals may be thrown into a homosexual panic by contact with an overt homosexual. Retarded in psychosexual development, the homosexual patient is confused by a heterosexual society and his behavior reflects this confusion. Everyone supposedly has the ability to be bisexual (sexually satisfied by men or women) but homosexuality is considered a normal behavior pattern only during the latency stage of development.

PSYCHODYNAMICS

Early in life a child needs to develop some degree of gender identity, or some idea of himself as a boy or girl, according to the expectations of the group he lives in.

Culture has encouraged feminine girls and masculine boys as the culture defines these adjectives. For some children, their conflicts over the sexual role may continue in adult life as unsureness about gender.

The adult may overcompensate and try to seduce everyone in sight. The Don Juan and the frigid flirt are not really interested in either sex or in the opposite sex. They are trying to prove their masculinity and femininity. Such over-compensation may also be non-sexual. The dictator and the martyr show exaggerated masculine-feminine attributes.

The adult may also act out his desire to be a different sex in socially acceptable ways. A man may marry a strong dominant woman and play the passive dependent role. A woman may take the dominant position at home or be a civic leader outside the home.

Such confusions do not always involve sex, but when they do, they favor the development of deviations, especially homosexuality. All the deviations or behaviors involving more than one person may be either heterosexual or homosexual and all are "normal" at some stage of development. They suggest arrested sexual development and adaption at the Oedipal and sometimes the anal stage.

Sado-masochism arises from experience with physical stimulation and skin contact and unresolved castration fear. Voyeurism is quite common in childhood. Fetishism is displayed in many activities from shooting toy guns to cuddling stuffed animals.

In addition to being in a state of arrested development, the sexual deviate has a weak ego and has never trusted his own worth or autonomy.

The rapist's ego is so weak he cannot even attempt to function sexually with another individual for fear of rejection. He uses force. Currently, rape is considered an act of violence, not a sexual behavior.

The pedophiliac cannot even manage intercourse with an adult, his weak ego can cope with nothing more threatening than a child.

The parent who commits incest with his child has an even weaker ego. He cannot even approach a strange child for fear of rejection; he approaches his own child in his own home.

The necrophiliac goes further. His ego cannot cope with anything more threatening than a dead body. The voyeur can only watch; and the fetishist can cope only with inanimate objects.

All of these behaviors are overt and observable. In contrast the homosexual may be latent and attempt to hide his homosexuality. Or, he may be bisexual and maintain a heterosexual relationship and a homosexual relationship at the same time or alternately.

Many individuals split the sexual from the romantic in their interpersonal relationships. A man may enjoy women sexually but his romantic attachments are to men. He doesn't really like women. If he does get involved with them he's angry and hurt and rejects them. He tries to avoid women except for sex; his real pleasure is in the company of men. The same thing is true of women. There are women who relate to men well sexually but don't like men; they resent men, compete with them, and are much happier and more affectionate with women.

The person who is wholly overtly homosexual has no desire to change and organizes his life around his sexual orientation. Overt homosexuals differ in dynamic organization. Some homosexual men are effeminate and may prefer to be treated like women. Others are masculine in attitudes and feelings but sexual desires are for men.

As more research is done (and homosexuality is a favorite problem for research) opinions may change. Although some theorists feel that the majority of homosexuals have no clear-cut or exclusive preference for active or passive roles, a recent study (Haist) seemed to support the "butch-fem" dichotomy, with the inserters preferring an active/masculine role and the insertees showing passive/feminine preferences in social situations.

Bullough views homosexuality as submissive (the active member having feelings of supremacy as of conquering the other) with anal intercourse involving hostility but the oral-genital contacts devoid of hostile implications.

The same is true of homosexual women, some are masculine, some feminine, but their sexual desires are for women.

The masculine woman and feminine men are the homosexual stereotypes. But what of the others?

1. The feminine homosexual woman feels like a woman but can't stand a penis so she chooses a masculine woman for her partner. In essence, she has found a castrated male. She has a strong castrating feeling and strong inhibition against male sexuality.
2. The masculine man feels active and aggressive as a man but hates women and especially their genitals, so he seeks passive homosexual males. The fear of castration is provoked by sight

of the "castrated" female genitalia and the vagina is viewed as a castrating instrument.

The child has two models of sexual behavior and he uses one (the same sex parent) to implement an action and the other (the opposite sex parent) to anticipate reaction. He sees and reacts to his parents' actions and the reaction of the child is more important than the actual act of the parents. Some children reject their parents because of the parents' heterosexual activities. Lesbians see heterosexual sex as sado-masochistic and are afraid of being injured by the penis. They rebel against their mothers, have problems competing with other women and a need for maternal comfort in their relationship with others.

During the Oedipal stage, homosexuals did not make the needed transfer from one parent to the other. The girl never gave up her mother to want her father. The boy did not want to win his mother. Perhaps these behaviors were due to fear or to some other phenomenon but whatever the cause, the homosexual is inherently immature and incapable of having a close adult relationship with a member of the opposite sex.

NURSING INTERVENTIONS

The sexual deviant is difficult to help. He responds to therapy slowly, if at all. Rarely is he a patient for treatment of his homosexuality, therefore his homosexuality is of importance only as a behavior indicative of developmental retardation. Be firm but kind, accept him as a person. Show him the same respect and concern as any other patient. Set limits, intervene in overt acts towards others and clarify the difference between acceptable behavior within a specific group (fellow homosexuals) and within a diverse group (patient unit). He has his rights but other patients also have theirs.

Avoid being manipulated and invited to converse in or to understand his "code" words. He will sometimes need protection from others (in panic or just annoyed) and others need to be protected from his more inappropriate behaviors. Rarely does he need physical care and recreational activities can be whatever he wishes, although neither body contact sports nor dancing with patients of the same sex is helpful.

If the behavior of the opposite sex parent has been identified, it helps not to repeat the behavior in relating to the patient. Avoid showing disgust, contempt, or fear.

Attitudes are important aspects of any relationship. Homosexuality has been viewed as a sickness, then as a deviation, and more recently as a personal life-style that concerns only those involved.

Nurses have their own problems and view homosexuality with interest, horror, disgust, indifference, sympathy, understanding or agreement - depending upon their own backgrounds and life-styles.

Deviant patients may become "too familiar" with the nurse, asking for personal information, dates, or making physical advances. Since most psychiatric patients have difficulties in personal relationships, the nurse should carefully explore the meaning of the behavior for the patient - the advances may indicate a healthy movement toward more mature relationships - or it may be that the patient is reacting to the nurse's behavior in a way he believes she wants him to respond. The nursing approach to these behaviors is similar to that with medical-surgical patients. If the behavior is verbal, the nurse should:

1. Be nonresponsive to the covert content.
2. Explore what his advances mean to him.
3. Ask patient what the personal information (date or advance) would mean to their lives.
4. Seek to uncover the feelings the flirtatious behavior masks:
   a. if the patient fears dependency, help him find ways to be more independent.
   b. if he fears the nurse will not provide him care without flirting, re-establish a mature relationship with him that does not require personal flattery.
   c. if he needs to manipulate, intervene as previously described.
   d. if he feels his manhood is threatened, explore verbally.

If the patient makes physical contact with the nurse, the best approach is to:

1. Request the patient not to touch her, saying that his actions make her feel uncomfortable.
2. Have patient put into words what he was thinking when he acted as he did.
3. Help bring his anxiety to the surface and reduce the anxiety as previously described.

Many patients who are hospitalized for some time masturbate, a behavior that may cause nurses and staff to withdraw and avoid him. This may cause more guilt and anxiety in the patient and he masturbates more, setting up the familiar pattern of mutual withdrawal. Masturbation may be an attempt to reach out to others, and is often done by people who are lonely, and denied their usual sexual outlets. Patients who forget in their anxiety that the observer may find such behavior threatening should be reminded that public masturbation makes others uncomfortable and request they limit masturbation to private times, as done with adolescents.

Psychiatric nurses conducting one-to-one therapy sometimes have sexual overtures made toward them, not as an expression of love but as resistance to therapy. Sexual acting-out may also be due to transference factors, as frequently encountered with schizophrenic patients.

Much has been written about the adverse effect that nurses who are disgusted by deviant behavior (homosexuality being only one of the deviant behaviors) have upon a patient's self-esteem and ability to cope positively. Women involved in rape and abortion cases have been treated as unworthy of care. Alcoholics and drug addicts have been shunned and ignored. But little is written about the other problem attitudes. Homosexuality is not unknown among psychiatric nurses (nor is alcoholism, abortion or drug addiction) and identifying with the patient, establishing a relationship with homosexual overtones or openly soliciting patients is no more therapeutic than ignoring or despising them.

An overt homosexual (patient or nurse) involved in the everyday life of a unit can cause homosexual panic in latent homosexuals and great unrest in other patients as well.

Women are thought to be latent (unconscious) homosexuals by tradition, although they may be merely "homosocial" (social relationships with women). Men are assumed to be overt (active, conscious) homosexuals more often than latent and society has traditionally viewed lesbians (female homosexuals) with more tolerance than it has viewed the male homosexual.

Perhaps that is why lesbians may provoke acute anxiety states and chronic uneasiness but latent male homosexuals may be thrown into violent homosexual panics when forced into close relationships with other men. Behaviors in panic are extreme agitation, ideas of reference (projecting own thoughts onto others and reacting to them), perplexity, hallucinations, paranoid delusions, may attack those men whom he feels are going to attack him sexually.

The patient needs help in controlling himself and may become violent if forced to remain in the threatening situation. He needs to be removed from frightening contacts until he can function more adequately. Don't assume that all patients or staff who respond negatively to the homosexual patient are latent homosexuals. Homosexuals can be childish, demanding, obnoxious - behaviors unrelated to his deviation. Reactions may be to his inadequacy in interpersonal relationships rather than to his sexual threat.

Deviant patients frequently have passive-aggressive behaviors, expressing their hostility indirectly by sulking, procrastinating and being stubborn rather than directly expressing feelings. These noncompliant behaviors often evolve from excessive parental demands which the child learns to deal with in subtle devious ways that permit him to avoid open conflict with authority. He pouts, inwardly resenting but unable to rebel openly.

The first step in the approach is to identify the pattern; hypothesis can be tested by structuring situations to see if the person complies with requirements. Once the hypothesis is confirmed, the following steps are suggested (Dixson):

1. Direct, matter of fact confrontation.
2. Setting specific limits which are enforced.
3. Discussing alternative behaviors.
4. Presenting consequences.
5. Providing opportunities for passive-aggressive person to verbalize negativism and anger.

6. Consistent, immediate follow-up of consequences.
7. Exploring connection between feeling of resentment and passivity.

The nurse's basic task with the deviant patient is to face her own inclinations and attitudes to prevent their interfering with the nurse-patient relationship. Physical care is rarely needed and close care is avoided along with recreational activities calling for close body contact. The patient may need to be protected from other patients as well as prevented from interfering with them. Communication is rarely difficult but using "code" words and the homosexual vocabulary may lead to personal involvement.

REVIEW QUESTIONS

1. What is sexual deviation?
2. Define some of the behaviors seen in sexual deviation.
3. How can sexual deviation be prevented?
4. Why is homosexuality considered deviant?
5. At what level of development are sexual deviants arrested?

SUGGESTED REFERENCES

1. Aaron, W.: Straight, Bantam Books, New York, 1972

2. Adams, G.: Recognizing the Range of Human Behavioral Sexism, Am J Maternal Child Nursing III:166-175, May-June, 1976

3. Addelso, F.: Induced Abortion: A Source of Guilt or Growth?, Am J Psychi XLIII, 1975

4. Barlow, D.H., et al.: Gender Identity Change in a Transsexual, Arch Gen Psychi, pp. 569-576, April, 1973

5. Bengis, I.: Combat in the Erogenous Zone, Bantam Books, New York, 1972

6. Bernard, F.: An Enquiry Among a Group of Pedophiles, J Sex Research XI:242-255, Aug., 1975

7. Bracken, M.B., et al.: The Decision to Abort and the Psychological Sequelae, J Nervous Mental Disorders, pp. 154-161, Feb., 1974

8. Braneman, S.: Homosexuality, Am J Nursing CXXIII:632-655, April, 1973

9. Bullough, V.: Sex and the Medical Model, J Sex Research XI: 291-303, Nov., 1975

10. Callahan, E.J. and Leitenberg, H.: Aversion Therapy for Sexual Deviation, J Abnormal Psychol LXXXI:60-75, Feb., 1973

11. Dannels, J.C.: Homosexual Panic, Perspectives Psychi Care X:106-111, Sept., 1972

12. Garrett, T. and Wright, R.: Wives of Rapists and Incest Offenders, J Sex Research XI:149-157, May, 1975

13. Gibney, H.A.: Masturbation: An Invitation for an Interpersonal Relationship, Perspectives Psychi Care X:128-134, Sept., 1972

14. Gordon, D., Ed.: Sex Games That People Play, Ace Books, New York, 1970

15. Green, R.: Homosexuality as a Mental Illness, International J Psychi X:77-98, March, 1972

16. Haist, M. and Hewitt, J.: The Butch-Fem Dichotomy in Male Homosexual Behavior, J Sex Research X:68-74, Feb., 1974

17. Hatterer, L.J.: Changing Homosexuality in the Male, McGraw-Hill Book Co., New York, 1970

18. Hoffman, M.: The Gay World, Bantam Books, New York, 1968

19. Johnston, J.: Lesbian Nation, Simon & Schuster, New York, 1973

20. Karlen, A.: Sexuality and Homosexuality, W.W. Norton, New York, 1971

21. Kroah, J.: How to Deal with Patients who Act Out Sexually, Nursing 1973, pp. 38-39, Dec., 1973

22. LeVine, W.R. and Barnstein, P.E.: Is the Sociopath Treatable? The Contribution of Psychiatry to a Legal Dilemma, University Law Quarterly, Vol. IV, Washington, 1973

23. McCaffrey, J.A., Ed.: The Homosexual Dialectic, Prentice-Hall, Englewood Cliffs, N.J., 1972

24. Mims, F. (Guest Editor): Human Sexuality, The Nursing Clinics of North America, Part II, 1975

25. Money, J.: Sexology: Behavioral, Cultural, Hormonal, Neurological, Genetic, etc., J Sex Research IX:3-10, Jan., 1973

26. Panken, S.: The Joy of Suffering, Jason Aronson, Inc., New York, 1973

27. Reuben, D.: Everything You Always Wanted to Know About Sex, Bantam Books, New York, 1969

28. Robertiello, R.C.: One Psychiatrist's View of Female Homosexuality, J Sex Research IX:30-33, Feb., 1973

29. Schafer, S.: Sexual and Social Problems of Lesbians, J Sex Research XII:50-69, Feb., 1976

30. Schaltz, L.G.: Child Sex Victims: Social, Psychological, and Legal Perspectives, Child Welfare 52:148-154, March, 1973

31. Seigelman, M.: Parental Background of Homosexual and Heterosexual Women, Br J Psychi CXXIV:14-21, Jan., 1974

32. Ujhely, G.: Two Types of Problem Patients and How to Deal with Them, Nursing 1976 VI:64-67, May, 1976

33. Van Den Aardweg, G.: A Grief Theory of Homosexuality, Am J Psychother XXVI:55-68, Jan., 1972

34. Woods, R.: Violence: Psychotherapy of Pseudohomosexual Patients, Arch Gen Psychi, Aug., 1972

35. Widom, C.S.: Interpersonal Conflict and Cooperation in Psychopaths, J Abnormal Psychol III:85-94, June, 1976

CHAPTER 12

THE CHILD WITH EMOTIONAL DISTURBANCES

The committee on Child Psychiatry of the Group for the Advancement of Psychiatry has proposed the following classifications of psychological disorders in children (GAP):

1. Healthy Responses
2. Reactive Disorders
3. Developmental Deviations
4. Psychoneurotic Disorders
5. Personality Disorders
6. Psychotic Disorders
7. Psychophysiologic Disorders
8. Brain Syndromes
9. Mental Retardation
10. Other Disorders

Healthy responses involve developmental or situational crises such as separation anxiety, grief, and clinging behavior.

Reactive disorders depend less on the severity of the stimuli than upon the child's reactions and ability to cope. Reactive disorders are most common in infants and preschoolers and include anaclitic depression, thumb-sucking, and withdrawn behavior.

Developmental deviations may involve total maturational deviation or include delayed, uneven, or exceptional patterns of motor, sensory, affective, social, psychosexual, cognitive, integrative, or speech development. Behaviors exhibited include low frustration tolerance, impulsivity, and prelogical thought processes.

Psychoneurotic disorders result when sexual and aggressive impulses are repressed and remain unresolved with resultant conflicts. These disorders rarely occur before school age. The child's unconscious conflicts cause anxiety; they react to the danger by forming symptoms to deal with the conflict symbolically. The types of disorders are the same as in the adult: anxiety, phobias (school), conversion (motor tics), dissociative (amnesia), obsessive-compulsive (rituals, orderliness), depressive (suicide).

Personality disorders manifest as fixed pathological traits such as isolation, dependence, impulsivity, and in behaviors such as glue sniffing, aggression, suspicion.

Psychophysiologic disorders refer to psychosomatic disorders such as asthma, migraine, ulcerative colitis, eczema, epilepsy and obesity.

Brain syndromes may be minimal to severe, acute or chronic. Severe chronic syndromes include cerebral palsy and inborn metabolic errors. Severe acute syndromes include alcohol intoxication, poison, or drugs. Minimal brain damage may manifest as hyperactivity, learning difficulties, impulsivity, perceptual problems or poor coordination. The syndrome may be almost unnoticeable but the child usually has just enough developmental lag to be considered slow by his peer group. The child may react by regressing, withdrawing, clowning, and developing a poor self-concept with low self-esteem. The adolescent with minimal brain damage has the usual tasks/independence, basic work skills, peer relationships, and sexual identity to master but even more difficulty in maturing. Drug addiction is rare but this adolescent is more prone than others of his age to become delinquent.

Mental retardation refers to subaverage general intellectual functioning associated with impaired adaptive behavior. Arising during the developmental period, mental retardation may be biological (known etiology such as trauma or chromosomes), environmental (psychosocial deprivation), or intermediate (both biological and environmental such as sensory organ defects). Mentally retarded children, adolescents, and/or adults may have the same problems of adjustment that other individuals do. They may be neurotic or psychotic, young or old, male or female. They have varying personalities and varying capabilities. Mental retardation is not a disease, nor is it a mental health problem. Mental retardation describes present behavior, without predicting potential.

The psychotic disorders are manifested in extreme, pervasive deviations in behavior. The child is aloof, preoccupied with inanimate objects, has outbursts of panic, bizarre stereotyped behavior patterns. He has a poor sense of personal identity and severely impaired interpersonal relationships. These are the children most often recognized as emotionally disturbed.

Infantile autism and childhood schizophrenia are sometimes viewed as separate disorders, sometimes as parts of the same illness. Autism occurs in infancy before development of a separate identity or ego; schizophrenia occurs later in childhood and is a regression to the infantile level. There may be evidence of organic brain damage in some of these children.

OVERT BEHAVIOR

Autistic children withdraw from the world and from reality and have severe problems with establishing a separate identity. They receive impressions through all their senses but cannot seem to "process" the information correctly. They are sometimes so unresponsive to stimuli they may appear deaf. Communication problems are universal in autistic children. All the behaviors may exist in varying forms and varying intensities. The child may display such behaviors as:

1. Sleeping and eating disturbance.
2. Bowel or bladder incontinence.
3. Repetitive stereotyped behavior.
4. Withdrawal.

5. Sensitivity to light, sound, and touch.
6. Severe tantrums.
7. Self-destructive behavior (headbanging, biting self, scratching self).
8. Aggression, especially against inanimate objects, destroys objects without seeming purpose or discrimination.
9. Enjoys TV commercials but not programs.
10. Likes things that can be turned or twirled (knobs, sticks, etc.).
11. Lack of emotion or "inappropriate" emotions.
12. Communication problems may range from no speech, through gibberish, to infantile speech patterns. No matter what level of language is attained, the content has little communicative value until "translated". Refers to self in third person.
13. Can't identify own body parts or define body limits. Doesn't know where his hands are in relation to his body. Will use another person's hands as extensions of his own.
14. Bizarre behavior - rocking, headbanging, "normal activities" performed with inappropriate affect.

PSYCHODYNAMICS

The early mother-child relationship is a symbiotic one (symbiosis meaning a close association necessary to one or both and not harmful to either). Only through the mother does the child begin identifying his ego boundaries, his body, and his identity. He is completely dependent upon his mother and finds the relationship frightening. Yet when his ego is just developing, he learns to walk, and moves away from his mother. He is filled with panic as he feels his ego threatened with total destruction.

If he cannot restore the relationship, he cannot maintain his ego development and regresses to that time when he did have complete possession of his mother - the symbiotic period.

The new relationship is closer to parasitism, in which close association is harmful to one or both of the members. The child is afraid to develop for fear of losing self or mother (to him the same thing), or to regress further for fear of being completely "smothered" by the mother. He has to control the degree of symbiosis and uses most of his energy in magic rituals and maneuvers to keep his mother at just the right distance.

His ego boundaries once again include his mother and he can't differentiate the "me" from the "not me". He can't perceive of his body as a whole, and may regard his body as an extension of his mother's, or his mother's body as an extension of his. He denies not only internal and external stimuli, responding with neither action nor emotion, he also denies his separate identity. In early infantile autism, the child includes everything and doesn't know where he ends and the world begins. The older child excludes himself from everything and has nothing left to distinguish himself from. Neither child can identify himself in time or space except in relationship to others, and has problems in "being". He may not know if he is a boy or girl, a human being, or a chair.

Aside from a weak ego, the autistic child's condition may involve specific family dynamics. One parent may have severe psychological problems while the other parent supports and depends upon the sick one. Often a complete inability to define roles exists within the family structure with resultant inconsistent behavior in the area of gender identity. Mother may be dependent, guilty, and view the child as an extension of herself, expressing the wish for the child to be "good" and make up for her own "badness". The father may be weak, rigid, often absent.

The family interactions may be cold, superficial, and filled with un-expressed hostility and jealousy. Although many authorities stress the family responsibility in producing an autistic child, others consider biological factors may be causative (excessive catecholamines for example). Still others emphasize the dynamic ego function. Probably autism and schizophrenia are produced from multiple causes, no one factor being sufficient in itself to produce abnormality.

NURSING INTERVENTIONS

The nurse working with psychotic children needs knowledge in at least three areas:

1. Normal growth and development.
2. Psychiatric therapeutic techniques.
3. Her own "hang-ups".

As a member of the psychiatric team, the nurse helps in assessing and evaluating the child.

Observation and communication are essential skills needed to interview the child and his family and to assess the nursing problems. In order to evaluate accurately, certain information is needed:

1. General appearance: Stage of development, abnormalities, affect, attitude, clothing.
2. Motor function: Degree of activity, abilities, walk, dexterity, abnormalities.
3. Communication pattern: Extent and use of language, expressiveness, content, body language, object of communication, length, general affect, some estimate of intelligence.
4. Emotional state: Emotions expressed (fear, rage, joy, apathy) and the appropriateness of emotion relative to the rest of the situation involved.
5. Identity and body image: Does he know body parts? Can he identify himself and others separately? Refers to himself in first person or third?
6. Interpersonal relationships: Is he withdrawn or aggressive? Does he relate to people or treat people as objects? Does he keep a large space between self and others or sit close to specific individuals, etc.?
7. General behavior: Bizarre? Compulsive? Withdrawn? Aggressive?

In addition it is necessary to observe the child's:

1. Sleeping and eating habits
2. Toilet training
3. Self-help abilities

The first intervention is to establish some form of communication. Observations of the child's developmental stage and his approach to others will help in communicating. Sometimes non-verbal language is the first contact with a withdrawn child and physical control the first contact with an aggressive child.

Once communication is established, a relationship may be developed. The primary intervention is actually an educational one: helping the child master the next developmental task.

The withdrawn child may have to learn to talk to others, to use language to satisfy some of his needs. The aggressive child needs immediate control to prevent injury to himself or to others. Behavior needs to be observed closely to identify patterns that signal a breakdown in control. The nurse needs to know what the precipitating behavior is in order to prevent violence, the child needs to identify his behavior in order to control it.

Children can be worked with easily through play, story telling, painting, poetry or music. Any approach to the child is governed by his developmental level, his ability to function, his present emotional state, and the nurse's skill and personality. The priorities in intervention are:

1. Physical care
2. Safety
3. Communication
4. Re-education

It is possible to change the child's behavior through the simple process of imitation. Almost any child will imitate someone close to him. He can learn language and simple behaviors by imitating the nurse who works with him.

The nurse's basic task is to help the child progress to the next developmental stage. She communicates through nonverbal actions, talks when the child is ready to hear, and listens always. The disturbed child needs physical care and protection from himself as well as from others. Safety is a top priority with these children. Activities are educational and utilized for fun, for growth, and for re-education. Whether the child is neurotic, psychotic, or mentally retarded, he is a child, whose primary need is to work through the developmental stages and establish his self-identity.

REVIEW QUESTIONS

1. How do infantile autism and childhood schizophrenia differ?
2. What are some of the overt behaviors demonstrated by autistic children and how can they be changed?

3. Is schizophrenia more environmental or more genetic?
4. What is the relationship of the schizophrenic child to his mother?
5. What things does a nurse need to know in order to work with autistic children?
6. Is observation of any help in evaluating an autistic child? Why or why not?
7. How can the aggressive child be controlled?

SUGGESTED REFERENCES

1. Allen, F.H.: Positive Aspects of Child Psychiatry, W.W. Norton & Co., New York, 1963

2. Barten, H. and Barten, S.S., Ed.: Children and Their Parents in Brief Therapy, Behavioral Publications, New York, 1973

3. Bender, L.: The life course of children with schizophrenia, Am J Psychi CXXX:783-788, 1973

4. Bettelheim, B.: The Children of the Dream, The Macmillan Co., New York, 1969

5. Bettelheim, B.: Love is Not Enough, The Free Press, Glencoe, Ill., 1950

6. Bettelheim, B.: The Empty Fortress, The Free Press, Glencoe, Ill., 1967

7. Bishop, B.R.: A new look for the psychiatric nurse: The child-care specialist, Perspectives Psychi Care XI:17-19, 1973

8. Chapman, A.H.: The Games Children Play, Berkley Publishing Corp., New York, 1971

9. Ekstein, R.: Children of Time and Space, of Action and Impulse, Appleton-Century Crofts, New York, 1966

10. Gardner, R.A.: MBD The Family Book About Minimal Brain Dysfunction, Jason Aronson, Inc., New York, 1973

11. Gardner, R.A.: Understanding Children, Jason Aronson, Inc., New York, 1973

12. Gardner, R.W. and Moriarty, A.: Personality Development at Preadolescence, University of Washington Press, Seattle, 1968

13. Graliker, B., et al.: Initial reactions and concerns of parents to a diagnosis of MR, Pediatrics XXIV:819-821, Nov., 1959

14. Group for the Advancement of Psychiatry: Psychological Disorders in Childhood, Jason Aronson, New York, 1974

15. Hamblin, R.L., et al.: The Humanization Process: A Social, Behavioral Analysis of Children's Problems, John Wiley & Sons, Inc., New York, 1971

16. Harrison, S.L. and McDermott, J.F., Ed.: Childhood Psychopathology, International Universities Press, New York, 1972

17. Hyde, N.: Behavior therapy in mental retardation, Am J Nursing V:881-885, May, 1974

18. Johnson, O. and Bommarito, J.: Tests and Measurements in Child Development: A Handbook, Jossey-Bass, Inc., San Francisco, 1971

19. Kammerman, S.B., et al.: Research and Advocacy, Children Today I:35-36, March-April, 1972

20. Kessler, J.W.: Neuroses in children, Manual of Child Psychopathology, Wolman, B.B., Ed., McGraw-Hill Book Co., New York, pp. 387-435, 1972

21. Kolstoe, O.: Mental Retardation, Holt, Rinehart & Winston, Inc., New York, 1972

22. Laury, G.: Psychotherapy with glue sniffers, International J Child Psychother I:98-110, 1972

23. Laybourne, P.C. and Churchill, S.W.: Symptom discouragement in treating hysterical reactions of childhood, International J Child Psychother I:111-123, July, 1972

24. Mussen, P.H., Ed.: Carmichael's Manual of Child Psychology, John Wiley & Sons, Inc., New York, 1970

25. Report of the Joint Commission on Mental Health of Children: 1. Crisis in Child Mental Health, 1969; 2. Mental Health: From Infancy Through Adolescence, 1973, Harper & Row, New York

26. Robinson, H.B. and Robinson, N.M.: The Mentally Retarded Child, McGraw-Hill Book Co., New York, 1965

27. Satir, V.: Peoplemaking, Science and Behavior Books, Inc., Palo Alto, Calif., 1972

28. Segal, J., Ed.: The Mental Health of the Child, U.S. Government Printing Office, Washington, D.C., 1971

29. Solnit, A.J. and Stark, M.H.: Mourning and the birth of a defective child, Psychoanalytic Study of the Child XVI:523-537, 1961

30. Szurek, S.A. and Berlin, I.N., Eds.: The Antisocial Child, His Family and His Community, Science and Behavior Books, Palo Alto, Calif., 1969

31. Thomas, A., et al.: Temperament and Behavior Disorders in Children, N.Y. University Press, New York, 1968

32. Ward, S.A.: Components of a child advocacy program, Children Today I:38-40, March-April, 1972

33. Whitaker, J.K. and Trieschman, A.E.: Children Away From Home, Aldine-Atherton, Chicago, 1972

34. Wolfe, S.: Children Under Stress, Penguin Press, London, 1969

35. Wooley, D.W.: The Biochemical Bases of Psychoses, John Wiley & Sons, Inc., New York, 1962

36. Wolman, B.: Children Without Childhood, Grune & Stratton, New York, 1970

37. Wolman, B.B.: Manual of Child Psychopathology, McGraw-Hill Book Co., New York, 1972

38. Woltman, A.G.: Puppetry as a tool in child psychotherapy, International J Child Psychother I:84-96, Jan., 1972

CHAPTER 13

THE ADOLESCENT WITH ADJUSTMENT PROBLEMS

Psychological adolesence begins with the growth spurts and bodily changes associated with puberty. Adolescence is successfully completed when the adolescent has formulated a stable personal and sexual identity, has a commitment to employment, a workable set of values and ethics, the ability to make decisions and solve his own problems and has established effective, interpersonal relationships with members of the opposite sex (GAP Report).

The "normal" adolescent displays behavior which can be considered abnormal or psychotic if viewed alone. The behavior has to be evaluated in the context of his personal life style, and the environmental influences. If his behavior is frankly schizophrenic, he resembles the adult more than the child in both behavior and care.

He may also continue somatic behaviors begun in childhood such as obesity, colitis, ulcers, and allergies. He may be involved in any of the neurotic responses to anxiety: phobia, obsession, compulsion, conversion.

Usually the adolescent has problems when his adaptive behavior becomes unrealistic and ineffective but not overtly psychotic. He may become antisocial, delinquent, or he may just daydream his way into trouble.

BODY IMAGE

Body image is the changing, evolving mental picture or psychological concept of one's body. Physical growth requires changes in one's body image and the rapid physical growth and sexual maturation of adolescence requires the successful re-orientation to the changing physical body. Self-identity previously established by body familiarity is weakened by the maturational changes and the chaotic adolescent period can be understood as a kaleidoscope of personality adjustments that take place from the period of latency to the emergence of a young adult. The awkward adolescent, ill at ease in his body, often unsure of where body parts extend, is greatly helped by physical activities such as sports and dancing. These help provide the vital "sense of where you are" in spatial terms. The recent societal emphasis on physical fitness has done much to aid the adolescent in successfully negotiating this difficult developmental life task.

The body image is the unique way each person has of perceiving his physical self, the unique concept each person holds of his own body as an object different from other objects. Combined with ego identity (the social self) the perception of the physical self shapes how one feels about oneself as a person. Disturbance in body imagery is an area of mutual concern to both neurologist and psychiatrist, since the body image is organized in the preconscious sensory motor cerebral cortex area. Kolb distinguishes these two disciplines' focus as the body image concept; the neurological body precept is the postural image one has of one's body as it functions outside of central consciousness, organized over the years and the result of tactile and kinesthetic perceptions. The body concept or conceptual, psychological image, includes perceptions, thoughts and feelings that the ego has in reference to viewing its own body. Failure of a person to perceive his body parts as they actually exist is most dramatically observed in the "phantom limb" phenomenon.

The body schema begins at birth and unfolds through interpersonal, environmental and body-ideal imagery. The maturing child gradually differentiates himself as a separate object from his mother. This progressive inclusion of body imagery in the child's mind is best measured by projective measures as the Draw A Person test, and predictive "norms" for body part drawings have been established.

Body boundaries are an important aspect of the body image concept. In the normal person, body boundaries coincide with the physical border of the body and body skin surface and body boundary are the same. When there are discrepancies between the actual body and the idealized "mental image" of the body, ego defenses may be formed to protect the person from the discrepancies. The "phantom limb" can be explained psychologically as a form of denial, and neurologically as memory traces at the subconscious level responding "as if" the receptor still existed.

Perceptions of body parts are on three levels: reality, conscious fantasy, and unconscious symbolic. Observations of the wide variations in adult medical-surgical patients to body-image alternating procedures illustrate the unique, unconscious symbolic meaning given to body parts by adults. Amputations, mastectomies, vasotomies, colostomies and rhinoplastic surgery may evoke severe body image disturbances. In working with adolescents who normally have body image discrepancies, or with medical-surgical patients, the nurse can often detect the beginning of body image problems by asking two questions:

1. Is the patient having strange body sensations?
2. Is the patient more aware of one body part than another?

Adolescents and adults can be diagnosed as having high or low body barriers, a distinction helpful for planning intervention. Women usually have higher body barriers than men, partly due to the "inside-outside" physical location of sexual organs. Female genitalia is internal and protected, while males' genitalia are "outside" the body, making them more vulnerable to body boundary problems. This is especially true for the male adolescent who can visually perceive sexual maturation.

High body barrier persons tend to perceive definite boundaries between their body and other objects, to be independent with low field-dependency. Low body barrier persons are more field dependent, rely more on peers for support (as juvenile gangs), and tend to attach their images to object possessions (as cars, motorcycles and belongings). Extreme forms of low body barriers are seen in the young schizophrenic who "depersonalizes", and delusionally attributes parts of his body and his thoughts to others. Unable to discriminate between external and internal body stimuli, his body and mind do not bind out what is felt, experienced, and perceived.

Small children naturally have weak ego boundaries, as can be observed in everyday life in their terrified reactions to having someone cut their hair or nails, body parts experienced as body boundaries. Schizophrenic children are often deficient in their body image, lacking in their ability to localize, discriminate and give meaning to mental images that need be integrated, clear in form and stable in time. Schizophrenia in adolescents may present in the severe affirmation of body boundaries, as seen in catatonic withdrawal; the lack of sensation in body parts due to the constricted posture, with a lack of sensory input a reversal of "phantom limb" phenomena.

The regression to a more childish level frequently seen in adolescence may also be due to the developing physical body and sex organs. These send out innumerable sensory stimuli and the adolescent becomes narcissistically preoccupied with himself in response to the continual sensory bombardment. Often he is unable to direct his energies outward. While his regression may be to the oral period, he has concurrent strivings for independence. Thus he substitutes objects for people to be dependent upon. The appeal of drugs and alcohol, the "object rather than person" vulnerability of the adolescent, can be explained, in part, as a maladaptive response to alterations in body images and self-concept.

The adolescent's autistic preoccupation with his body and its appearance is exploited by the "youth oriented" commercials, appealing to the greatest (unemployed) age group of spenders in our society. Insecure in the adequacy of changing body, the adolescent quickly succumbs to whatever "miracle" remedy is suggested. In the resurgence of orality, the adolescent's oral gratifications are usually in the form of a strangely unbalanced diet, causing "adolescent acne", the combined result of the excessive activity of the glandular system and parents' tendency to "MacDonald" their teenagers.

The extreme form of a dietary problem in adolescence is seen in the disorder termed anorexia nervosa. A misnamed emotional problem, the adolescent afflicted is underweight and emaciated, not due to a lack of appetite or affliction of the appetite center in the hypothalamus. These youngsters are usually frantically preoccupied with food yet have a dread of putting on too much weight. Their refusal to eat serves the ego and emphasizes oral traits. Characteristics of anorexia nervosa include:

1. Body image disturbances to delusional proportions, i.e., adolescent doesn't "see self" as thin and is bewildered by parental concern.
2. Normal stomach hunger sensations are repressed, denied (depersonalized) and not received on conscious level.
3. Feelings of ineffectualness and low sex drives predominate.

Other body image disturbances in anorexia nervosa include misconceptions of oral impregnation through food by unconscious symbolic ties between nurturing and food being rebelled against. Current diet fads and teenagers' concern for "body pollution" via preservatives and additives are other forms of "body image" rebellion. Both diet fads and anorexia nervosa can result in death - due to the irreversible metabolic processes set in motion.

Intervention in anorexia nervosa includes helping the adolescent reestablish connections between body sensations (hunger) and responses (eating). Since these defects are unconscious they respond to the opposite approach used in managing "phantom limb" desensitization, as the problems are but two sides of the same coin.

The adolescent, like the infant, also has great conflict over dependency and often exhibits the same ambivalence and negativism seen in the two-year-old. To emphasize "differences" between them and their parents, they closely identify with their peers, forming a counter-culture with exaggerated differences between generations. During the fifties, the generation gap was greatly extended since formal educational opportunities were available to children that their parents had not experienced. Never in the history of humanity had the youth more "formal learning" than the older generation. This fostered the decline in respect for the aged, student revolutions and "acting-out". A re-evaluation of knowledge versus wisdom followed (with the first astronauts "over forty"). Other social forces have intervened as the quest for equality superceded academic excellence, and the cognitive generation gap of the fifties and sixties is no longer an issue.

Adolescent recapitulation to childish patterns are also seen in the revival of the feelings of the Oedipal period. As in the first time around, identification with the parent of same sex is necessary and "flirtatious" relationships with that of opposite sex parent serve as preparation for later life. Opposite sex parents' approval is important reassurance to the adolescent, as daddy's approval gives the young girl the feeling she's acceptable. With maturation of sexual organs, the adolescent period is of lust. Masturbatory activity is generally considered normal, a preparation for heterosexual interpersonal contacts.

Parental reactions to the adolescent are of great significance. Parents may experience an oedipal resurgence (mid-forties). The parent of the same sex has a vital role as a "buffer" between the adolescent and parent of opposite sex. Acting as friend, providing "man-to-man" exchanges, or "girl talk", as often adolescents want to talk things over but make their own decisions. When parents do not provide for these exchanges, the youngsters may seek out identification with an older person parent substitute laying the seeds for homosexuality.

Concurrent to development of the sexual and physical image in adolescents is the establishment of high moral values and ethics; rap sessions, hours spent in peer talk, or on the telephone, help. The adolescent is critical of others, and has great self-criticism of his body as acceptable. Scrupulosity and religiosity as psychiatric symptoms may emerge at this time. Adolescents need freedom to experiment, opportunities to develop judgment from experience and to learn to cope.

Often heightened sexual drives merge with aggressive drives and result in suicide (due to moral values) or outward expression of aggression (vandalism). Suicide once was the leading cause of adolescent death; now adolescents, like their parents, control their aggressive-sexual drives by drugs. The tendency to self-medicate (drugs, alcohol and pot) has coincided with new "sexual freedom". Abortions and the pill provide a new liberated female adolescent.

OVERT BEHAVIOR

1. Defiant
2. Flippant
3. Sullen
4. Reluctant to talk about self but may converse extensively on irrelevant topics
5. Sexual deviations
6. Addiction to drugs or alcohol
7. Depression
8. Withdrawal
9. Testing and acting-out
10. Manipulative
11. Self-destructive

PSYCHODYNAMICS

Adolescence is a period of ambivalence. The adolescent wants to break away from his parents yet doesn't always feel sure enough of himself or independent enough to do so.

He wants close relationships with others yet often fears the competition of his peer group. He has great sexual drive yet fears failure or rejection in heterosexual relationships.

He wants to earn his own money, yet doesn't want to be responsible for earning his own living. He wants to be someone important but doesn't know how to accomplish it. He wants to save the world and can't solve his own internal conflicts.

He has to establish his identity as an individual, to integrate his past learnings, resolve his conflicts and emerge as a functioning adult.

Fantasy and daydreaming are ways of coping with his ambivalence. He possesses both a superior and an inferior concept of himself, but not one clear self-concept. He feels inferior because he has not been able to react to environmental stimuli in an effective manner but in his fantasies he can always emerge superior and victorious.

Like the daydreamer, the delinquent attempts to satisfy his desires without respect to reality. However, he is not satisfied with fantasy and resorts to acting out his demands.

Trying to exert his independence from adult values and authority, he becomes a willing "slave" to peer group pressures. He still does not have a true identity of his own for he identifies with gang standards and peer behavior.

The superego control is inadequate and id impulses are expressed openly. Stealing, murder, assault, malicious mischief are all ways to act-out his feelings that the world owes him a living.

Problems with gender identify arise from unresolved Oedipal conflicts and environmental stresses. He must prove himself a man by doing daredevil things and being active sexually. He never quite overcomes early feelings of inadequacy and the more he tries, the more chances for failure; the more failures, the less he feels like a man. The same processes occur in the adolescent girl, but her acting-out behavior may be confined to shoplifting and prostitution without the violent activities common in the boy's behavior.

An inability to establish an identity, to resolve conflicts, to master developmental tasks successfully may lead to anxiety, intense feelings of inferiority, deep depression, and eventual suicide (see Appendix A).

NURSING INTERVENTIONS

Communication

1. Set limits
2. Avoid being maternal, punitive, or judgmental
3. Refuse to be manipulated and point out his behaviors
4. Provide constructive experiences in interactions
5. Reinforce efforts to change
6. Help him identify the reality of his behavior

Physical Care

Rarely will the adolescent need physical care. He may need help with his appearance to avoid bizarre behavior. He may need positive reinforcement of appropriate diet habits and re-education for poor ones. If he is addicted to drugs or alcohol his physical care will depend upon his physical condition.

Protection

He needs protection from humiliation and embarrassment, but most of all he needs to be protected from his self-destructive impulses. Suicide is a real threat.

Recreation

He does better in groups. He needs gross motor activity to use up his excess energy but also needs creative opportunities. Sports, games, leather work, painting, sculpture, auto repair - are all excellent activities for the adolescent.

The adolescent sometimes relates better and responds faster to a young nurse who can be viewed as a peer. Others may do better with an older nurse who can give him the control he needs, yet accept him as he is.

The adolescent patient may be an antisocial personality, a drug addict or an alcoholic. He may be having withdrawal symptoms of DT's, or he may be lost in depression and contemplating suicide. He may be in a schizophrenic episode or phobic panic. Almost all behavior disorders of adults are manifested by adolescents.

The nurse's basic task with the adolescent is to help him master his developmental stage and progress to the next. He needs little physical care unless acutely ill, but much reassurance and support to motivate him to care for himself. He needs protection from his self-destructive urges, and recreational activities that will help him to grow and to understand himself a little better. The nurse can communicate easily if she avoids being manipulated and if she maintains control of any given situation.

The adolescent asks for help in many ways - but he does ask.

REVIEW QUESTIONS

1. What are the developmental tasks of adolescence?
2. What type of nurse would be most successful in dealing with the adolescent patient?
3. What are some of the behaviors observed and what do they mean?
4. What is "body image"?
5. Why is body image important in adolescence?

SUGGESTED REFERENCES

1. Aarons, Z.A.: Normality and abnormality in adolescence, Psychoanalytic Study of the Child XXV:309-339, 1970

2. Abernathy, V.: Sexual knowledge, attitudes, and practices of young female psychiatric patients, Arch Gen Psychi XXX:180-182, 1974

3. Anthony, J.S.: The reactions of parents to adolescents and to their behavior, In Parenthood: Its Psychology and Psychopathology, Anthony, J. and Benedek, T., Eds., Little, Brown & Co., Boston, pp. 307-324, 1970

4. Bardwick, J.M.: Psychological conflict and the reproductive system, Feminine Personality and Conflict, Belmont Books, Calif., pp. 3-28, 1970

5. Berkovitz, I., Ed.: Adolescents Grow in Groups, Brunner-Mazel, New York, 1972

6. Berne, E.: What Do You Say After You Say Hello, Bantam Books, New York, 1972

7. Blos, P.: The second individuation process of adolescence, Psychoanalytic Study of the Child XXII:162-186, 1967

8. Boyer, L.B.: A suicidal attempt by an adolescent twin, International J Psychoanalytic Psychother I:7-30, Aug., 1972

9. Boyer, C.M.: Caring for the young addict with tetanus, Am J Nursing LXXIV:265-267, Feb., 1974

10. Brown, D.G. and Lynn, D.B.: Human sexual development: An outline of components and concepts, J Marriage Family XXVIII: 155-162, 1966

11. Bruch, H.: Eating Disorders: Obesity, Anorexia Nervosa and the Persons Within, Basic Books, New York, 1973

12. Campion, E. and Tucker, G.: A note on twin studies, schizophrenia and neurological impairment, Arch Gen Psychi XXIX: 460-463, 741, 1973

13. Copel, S.L., Ed.: Behavior Pathology of Childhood and Adolescence, Basic Books, New York, 1973

14. Daedalus: Journal of American Arts and Sciences, Twelve to Sixteen: Early Adolescence, Fall, 1971

15. Dempsey, M.O.: The development of body image in the adolescent, Nursing Clinics N Am IV:609-615, Dec., 1972

16. Distler, L.S.: The adolescent "hippie" and the emergence of a matristic culture, Psychiatry XXXIII:362-371, 1970

17. Field, W.E. and Wilkerson, S.: Religiosity as a psychiatric symptom, Perspectives Psychi Care XI:99-105, 1973

18. Fisher, S.H.: Mechanisms of denial in physical disabilities, Arch Neurol Psychi, pp. 782-784, 1958

19. Fisher, S. and Cleveland, S.E.: Body Consciousness, Jason Aronson, New York, 1974

20. Group for the Advancement of Psychiatry: Normal Adolescence: Its Dynamics and Impact, Scribner, New York, 1968

21. Haggerty, R.J. and Rogers: Noncompliance and self-medication: Two neglected aspects of pediatric pharmacology, Ped Clinics N Am XIX:101-115, 1972

22. Hertzig, M.E. and Birch, H.G.: Neurological organization in psychiatrically disturbed adolescents, Arch Gen Psychi XIX: 526-536, 1976

23. Hudgens, R.W.: Psychiatric Disorders in Adolescents, The Williams & Wilkins Co., Baltimore, 1974

24. Jacobs, J.: Adolescent Suicide, Wiley Interservice, New York, 1971

25. Jurgensen, K.: Limit setting for hospitalized adolescent psychiatric patients, Perspectives Psychi Care IX:173-184, 1971

26. Kaufman, G. and Krupka, J.: Integrating one's sexuality: Crisis and change, International J Group Psychother XXIII:445-463, 1973

27. Kenniston, K.: Youth - A "new" stage of life, Am Scholar XXXIX:631-654, 1970

28. Kolb, L.C.: The body image in the schizophrenic reaction, Aver-Back, A., Ed., Schizophrenia, An Integrated Approach, Ronald Press, New York, 1959

29. Levinson, P.: Religious delusions in counter culture patients, Am J Psychi CXXX:136-139, 1973

30. Lorenz, K.: The enmity between generations and its probable etiological cause, Play and Development, Piers, M., Ed., W.W. Norton & Co., New York, 1972

31. Lynch, V.J.: Narcissistic loss and depression in late adolescence, Perspectives Psychi Care XIV:133-135, 1976

32. Masterson, J.F.: Treatment of the Borderline Adolescent: A Developmental Approach, J. Wiley & Sons, New York, 1972

33. Masterson, J.F.: The psychological significance of adolescent turmoil, Am J Psychi CXXIV:1549-1553, May, 1968

34. McCloskey, J.C.: How to make the most of body image theory in nursing, Nursing 1976 V:68-72, May, 1976

35. Meyer, H.: Predictable problems of hospitalized adolescents, Am J Nursing LXIX:525-528, March, 1969

36. Offer, D.: The Psychological World of the Teenager, Basic Books, New York, 1969

37. Peto, A.: Body image and archaic thinking, International J Psychoanal XL:223-231, 1959

38. Rachman, A.W.: Group psychotherapy in treating the adolescent identity crisis, International J Child Psychother I:97-119, 1972

39. Selvini, M.P.: Anorexia nervosa, Arieti, S., Ed.: The World of Psychiatry and Psychotherapy, Basic Books, New York, Vol. I, pp. 197-218, 1971

40. Shainess, N.: Is there a separate feminine psychology? NY State J Med LXX:3007-3009, 1970

41. Schilder, P.: The Image and Appearance of the Human Body, International University Press, New York, 1950

42. Sherrill, L.: Nursing the patient who expresses concern for self-identity, Perspectives Psychi Care II:30-34, March-April, 1964

43. Strutzel, E.A.: A disturbed adolescent: The nursing process in a collaborative treatment, Nursing Clinics N Am VI:727, Dec., 1971

44. Thomas, A. and Chess, S.: Evolution of behavior disorders into adolescence, Am J Psychi, pp. 509-524, 1976

45. Williams, J.: Intervention in maturational crisis, Perspectives Psychi Care VI:240-246, 1971

46. Winnicott, D.W.: Basis for self in body, International J Child Psychother I:7-16, 1973

47. Weiner, J.B.: Psychological Disturbance in Adolescence, Wiley-Interscience, New York, 1970

48. Zubin, J. and Freeman, A., Eds.: The Psychopathology of Adolescence, Grune & Stratton, New York, 1970

49. Roshin, S.: The adolescent in psychotherapy, Perspectives Psychi Care VII:263-266, 1969

CHAPTER 14

MIDDLE AGE AND INVOLUTIONAL MELANCHOLIA

The major life events of middle age include:

1. Reaching one's peak in a career
2. Launching children from the home
3. Death of parents
4. Climacterium
5. Grandparenthood
6. Illness (chronic and acute)
7. Retirement
8. Widowhood

There are no clear boundaries as to when middle age begins, as it is a psychological "state of mind" rather than a specific age span. Generally around 40, middle age begins; yet most men see no major differences before or after 40, while women report discontinuities in their lives "before and after" the mid-life mark. Perceptions of the life cycle are influenced by social values and change; currently our society worships youth, which, several decades ago was ignored. While current society is youth oriented, it is controlled by people who are middle aged, who generally report middle age as an exciting and rewarding life period. With better judgment and decision making mellowed by experience, most middle aged persons speak of being in the "prime of life". They are highly competent, preoccupied with self-utilization and see themselves as contributors to society. Healthy, well adjusted middle aged persons see middle age as an opportunity for growth and change, not stagnation. No longer driven, they frequently feel they are the "drivers", and at ease in their social positions.

Body changes during the middle years are more pronounced for men than for women. There is a personalization of death - with the fear of widowhood and heart attacks common. The major fear of both male and female middle aged persons, however, is the fear of dependency -- due to loss of income or loss of health (Garron). The fear intensifies as age increases.

Involution melancholia has been the "classical" psychiatric disease of the middle age life span. As most depressive diseases, it is more commonly found in females than males. Textbook distinctions between involutional melancholia and manic depressive illness specify that the involutional has:

1. No history of past episodes of depression
2. Rigid, obsessive-compulsive personality (not cyclothymic)
3. Gradual rather than abrupt onset
4. An absence of a manic state
5. Poor prognosis

Premorbid characteristics are a rigid adherence to an ethical code, a narrow range of interest, overmeticulousness, parsimony, stubborness, paranoia and poor sexual adjustment. The superego dominates the personality with anal erotic defenses of obsession-compulsions. The agitation and hyperactivity of the involutional is in marked contrast to other manic depressive disorders.

While the textbook pictures have become more detailed and refined in the disease description, the decrease in the number of diagnosed cases of involutional melancholia provides the eloquent discussion of involutional melancholia as a disappearing disease (Rosen). It is interesting to note that as diseases tend to disappear clinically, written descriptions become highly refined, as writings on the "vapors", chlorosis, and Febricula (Straus).

Unlike any other illness, mental illness is defined by time and place, subject to change by social definition and technological advances. Present changes in woman's role in society has had marked influence on the attitudes toward the climacterium and the involutional diagnosis. At one time, the end of the woman's productive period relegated her to the realm of the "unwanted". No longer considered a suitable sex object, her "life" was seen as over. Current attitudes toward the middle aged woman no longer casts her as a "has been". Recent research indicates that:

1. Instead of an ending, the psychic energy once given to menstrual and reproductive functions is now freed for the middle aged woman's psychological expansion (Benedict).
2. Females are most cognitively productive after menopause.
3. Child bearing and rearing experiences provide excellent preparation for larger social activities and involvements.
4. Women's sex drives continue and may even intensify after menopause since the unconscious fear of pregnancy may have inhibited sexual pleasure during the reproductive years (Masters and Johnson).
5. There is a growing body of evidence that the emotional problems of depressive syndromes are roughly correlated with MAO activity and hormonal replacement therapy is appropriate treatment (Grant).

With these constraints and changes in mind, the following textbook picture is presented.

The Middle Aged Involutional: Involutional psychoses were once considered to be part of the endocrine imbalance of the climacteric. Over the years, observations showed that many of the middle aged who demonstrated psychotic symptoms had similar personality patterns and similar precipitating experiences.

In the fifth and sixth decades of life (45 to 65), men and women are both faced with identity crises comparable to the ones faced in adolescence. The crises are more devastating because the past life is reviewed and found wanting, and there seems to be very little future left and even less hope.

In mild reactions, the middle aged individual may change jobs, up-rooting his entire family, have face-lifts, and other restitutive surgery, swap marriage partners, have extramarital relationships, turn to alcohol or drugs for comfort.

In severe psychotic reactions he may become depressed, paranoid, or both. No more profound depression exists than the involutional depression. Suicide is common. Paranoid delusions center around sex and authority rather than in the megalomania (or delusions of greatness: Christ, Caesar) of the paranoid.

OVERT BEHAVIOR

The depressive state:

1. Agitation, physical restlessness and pacing, crying, whining, and clinging, "picking" at skin or parts of body, early morning insomnia, loss of appetite and/or anorexia, and sexual deviation.
2. Repeated admissions of guilt and of having committed the "unpardonable sin", repeated statements of complete and total poverty, that everything is lost, and suicidal attempts.
3. Somatic delusions: Centering around the gastrointestinal system. Intestines are stopped up, stomach is "closed".
4. Nihilistic delusions: Express thoughts that the world no longer exists, that they are going to be left some place to die, that everything is empty and hell is beckoning.
5. Hallucinations: In keeping with the delusions, they may hear voices telling them to kill themselves, or not to eat food because they are going to die and no longer need it.

The paranoid state:

1. Agitation, aggression, anxiety, crying and clinging, physical restlessness, and jealousy.
2. Repeated complaints of sexual advances by others, exhibitionism.
3. Delusions of persecution - others are trying to destroy him.
4. Hallucinations in keeping with the delusional system.

PSYCHODYNAMICS

The premorbid personality of the typical involutional psychotic displays an anal compulsive orientation. Basic dependency needs were not met or satisfied in early childhood, but a strong superego keeps feelings of dependency, jealousy, and inadequacy under control.

Middle age involves physical changes that cannot be ignored. Facing both physical changes and environmental losses (job, friends, money, position) are too threatening and overwhelming for the super-ego to maintain control, and the energy is centered - not in the id - but in the ego. All forces are marshalled and focused on self and loss of self.

The loss of worth which is felt causes mourning or grief reactions which are openly displayed. The ego regresses to an oral dependency stage and the clinging dependent demands cannot be satisfied.

Some of the middle aged react to the changes as final and deadly and they have no hope for future resolution. Others can proceed from an acute break to complete recovery and live many more productive years.

The dynamics are much the same as for any depressive or paranoid state.

NURSING INTERVENTIONS

The depressive state:

1. Communication: Although it is difficult to break into such a severe depression, the nurse may be able to establish a relationship by first staying nearby and listening. Set limits on the number of times the admissions of the same guilt can be communicated; the repetition will not help him, controlling him may. Walk with him when he's pacing but try to distract him into another activity. Accept him as he is, not as he thinks he is. Identify his delusions and hallucinations as personal, don't enter into them. Support him but help him "grow" - don't reinforce his extreme dependency.

2. Physical care:
   a. Diet. May refuse to eat because he's dying or already dead and doesn't need it. Give frequent liquid snacks that fulfill nutritional as well as fluid requirements and keep intake and output records, especially a record of bowel movements. If the delusion of "stopped-up bowels" becomes reality, the patient's behavior will be strongly reinforced.
   b. Sleep. May be able to sleep for a few hours early in the night but awakens early and becomes restless. Try to keep him busy during the day and not in bed resting and keep him up as long as possible in the evening before midnight. If he has trouble falling asleep, physical measures (warm milk, back rubs, and warm baths) are soothing and satisfy some of his dependency needs.
   c. Skin. His skin will need care if he is apt to pick at it and cause lesions and possibly infection. His nutritional imbalance and lack of fluids may cause dry and cracking skin. Lotions are helpful. Manual activities to preoccupy him may lessen the agitated self-destruction.
   d. Appearance. He may consider the matter of appearance as irrelevant for one who is dead and need encouragement to bathe and dress appropriately. Usually he will be compulsively neat and clean, and need no help in dressing. The men will want to be shaved and can usually use an electric razor; the women may want to use their own cosmetics and do their own hair.

3. Protection: The involutional depressive needs protection against suicide. He may attempt suicide even in the depths of depression.

All care needs to be taken to ensure that he doesn't have any lethal weapons available (including mirrors, accumulated sleeping pills, unprotected windows), he is not isolated or out of sight for long periods, he is supported during threats or attempts, not dared or punished.

Sometimes, no matter what precautions are taken, a patient succeeds at suicide. No member of the psychiatric team need feel guilty or frustrated, but most members will.

4. Recreation: He needs to be with other people but is often rejected. Group activities without close interaction are less threatening than active participation in groups. Movies and group occupational therapy are better than competitive games or sports. His mind is clear and writing or painting may be therapeutic, as are other creative activities.

The paranoid state:

1. Communication: Difficult to establish a relationship with an extremely suspicious patient, especially when he is also an extremely dependent one. Clarify reality when a woman complains of sexual advances or "indecent gestures" from other patients, or when a man insists that his doctor and others in authority are spreading defamatory gossip about him. Set limits on complaining, "whining" behavior; try to provide distractors; accept and support him but avoid being manipulated; don't reinforce dependency needs; satisfy those that can be satisfied, and acknowledge others; point out that only he has the hallucination, and the delusions; don't enter into either one.
2. Physical care:
   a. Diet. May be too suspicious to eat, and wish to cook own food or eat with the nurse. More often he's too agitated to eat and can manage with finger foods from original packages. Needs chewable food more than liquids such as malts. Try to maintain adequate fluid intake.
   b. Sleep. Afraid to sleep with others. Try to give him a room by himself that is neither noisy enough to interfere with his sleep, nor so quiet that he hears and misinterprets every sound. Active physical measures to induce sleep may be threatening.
   c. Appearance. Usually has no problem maintaining his appearance, resents interference, would consider help as being a comment on his inferiority.
3. Protection: Other patients need to be protected from him but since depression exists in the paranoid state, suicide is always a threat. Needs close observation as unobtrusively as possible.
4. Recreation: Creative and manual tasks expend some of his energy and if he can play well enough to win, chess and other two-person activities may be beneficial. Avoid openly competitive games or sports in which his feelings of inadequacy will be reinforced. Any group activity may be threatening.

The nurse's basic task with the involutional patient is to establish an environment in which he can regain some self-respect and resolve his grief reactions from losses suffered. Physical care is necessary when depression is acute, and protection is needed to prevent both suicide and attacks on others. Activities are focused upon introducing him to group activities again, helping with creative endeavors, and avoiding open competition. Communication is difficult, limits have to be set on complaining and "whining", and hallucinations are identified but not entered into.

REVIEW QUESTIONS

1. Is there much difference in the behaviors manifested in the depressive and in the paranoid involutional state?
2. Do men have involutional problems?
3. How does the depressed behavior of the involutional patient differ from the behavior of the depressed patient?
4. Does the involutional patient need protection from others?
5. Will he do better with groups or alone?
6. How do you handle his delusion?
7. What would be some preventative measures to lessen the incidence of involutional psychosis?

SUGGESTED REFERENCES

1. Belbin, E. and Belbin, R.M.: New careers in middle age, In Neugarten, B.L., Middle Age and Aging, University of Chicago Press, Chicago, 1968

2. Benedek, T.: On the psychic economy of the developmental process, Arch Gen Psychi XVII:271-276, 1967

3. Berger, B.M.: The new stage of American man - Almost endless adolescence, New York Times Magazine, Nov. 2, 1969

4. Brown, C.W., et al.: Life events and psychiatric disorders: Part I: Some methodological issues, Psychological Med III:74-87, 1973

5. Clayton, P.J., et al.: The depression of widowhood, Br J Psychi CXX:71-77, 1972

6. Deynen, E.V., et al.: The empty nest - Psychosocial aspects of conflict between depressed women and their grown children, Am J Psychi CXXII:1422-1426, 1966

7. Dresen, S.: Adjusting to single parenting, Am J Nursing, pp. 1286-1289, Aug., 1976

8. Fried, E.: Does woman's new self-concept call for new approaches in group psychotherapy, International J Group Psychother, pp. 265-272, 1974

9. Frommer, E.A. and O'Shea, G.: Antenatal identification of women liable to have problems in managing their parents, Br J Psychi CXXIII:141-148, 1973

10. Garron, D.C.: Attitudes of middle aged persons toward growing older, Geriatrics VI:21-24, 1957

11. Grant, C. and Prepe-Davies, J.: Effects of oral contraceptives on depressive mood changes and on endometrial monoamina oxidase and phosphates, Br Med J XXVIII:777-780, 1968

12. Ginott, H.C.: Between Parent and Teenager, The Macmillan Co., Ontario, 1969

13. Havighurst, R.J.: Changing roles of women in middle years, In Gross, J., Ed., Potentialities of Women in the Middle Years, Michigan State University Press, 1956

14. Hellerstein, H.K. and Friedman, E.H.: Sexual activity and the post-coronary patient, Med Aspects Human Sexuality III:70-79, March, 1969

15. Kright, J.A.: The use and misuse of religion by the emotionally disturbed, Pastoral Psychol XIII:122-126, 1962

16. Marbach, A.H.: Sexual problems and gynecological illness, Med Aspects Human Sexuality IV:48-54, Dec., 1970

17. Mendels, J.: Concepts of Depression, John Wiley & Sons, New York, 1970

18. Miles, H.S. and Hays, D.: Widowhood, Am J Nursing LXXV: 280-284, Feb., 1975

19. Miller, J.B. and Molhner, J.: Psychological consequences of sexual inequality, Am J Orthopsychi XLI:767-775, 1971

20. Mushatt, C. and Werby, I.: Grief and anniversary reactions in a man of sixty-two, International J Psychoanalytic Psychother I:83-106, Nov., 1972

21. Myerson, P. and Aden, G., Eds.: Confrontations in Psychotherapy, Science House, New York, 1973

22. Neugarten, B.L.: Dynamics of transition of middle age to old age: Adaptation and the life cycle, J Geriatric Psychi IV:71-87, 1970

23. Porteores, H.: Sex and Identity, Bobbs-Merrill Co., New York, 1972

24. Pfeiffer, E., et al.: Sexual behavior in middle life, Am J Psychi CXXVIII:1262-1267, 1972

25. Rangell, L.: The return of the repressed oedipus, In Parenthood, Anthony, E.J. and Benedek, T., Eds., Little, Brown & Co., Boston, pp. 325-334, 1970

26. Rosen, S.: Involutional menucholia, In American Handbook of Psychiatry, Arieti, S., Ed., Basic Books, New York, 1974

27. Rozmoy, M.S.: How to take a sexual history, Am J Nursing LXXVI:1279-1282, Aug., 1976

28. Sachar, E.J., et al.: Disrupted 24-hour pattern of cortisol secretion in psychiatric depressions, Arch Gen Psychi XXVIII: 19-24, 1973

29. Sanborn, D.E. and Sanborn, C.J.: The psychological autopsy as a therapeutic tool, Diseases Nervous System XXXVII:4-8, 1976

30. Shapiro, D.A.: Symbiosis in adulthood, Am J Psychi CXXIX: 289-292, 1972

31. Shapiro, J.H.: Communities of the Alone, Association Press, New York, 1971

32. Soddy, K.: Men in Middle Life, Travistock, London, 1967

33. Spiegel, R.: Depressions and the feminine situation, In Goldman, G.D. and Milman, D.S., Eds., Modern Woman, Charles C. Thomas, Springfield, 1969

34. Straus, B.: Disappearing diseases, Med Counterpart, pp. 19-26, Feb., 1970

35. The involutional depressive syndrome, Am J Psychi, Supplement, pp. 21-35, May, 1968

CHAPTER 15

THE AGED AND SENESCENCE

Senility is partly organic and partly psychogenic. The aberrations in behavior are not directly related to the amount of organic change due to aging or to an arteriosclerotic episode. Organic damage to the brain is evidenced by changed behaviors in the three areas of memory, orientation, and judgment.

A schizophrenic may display problems in these areas, yet not be defective in any of them. He just doesn't care to say what day it is or where he is now.

The senile patient has actual defects and does not realize it. It is necessary to know the difference between actual defects and delusional systems.

For instance, if an elderly woman dresses up in an evening gown to go shopping, she might be either schizophrenic or senile. What is the difference? If she knows she's going shopping and still wears the gown, she's displaying poor judgment and is senile. If she thinks she is going to a premiere, she's using good judgment within her own delusional system and is psychotic.

If a man thinks he's in California and it's snowing outside, he is probably senile, but if he thinks he's a visiting dignitary on his way to see the President, he's delusional.

Many elderly people have defects in memory and orientation but they realize they're a little mixed up and react to and with the organic damage as best they can at the moment.

Some elderly people with organic brain damage react to the damage with psychotic behavior. They may become depressed, elated, delusional, or paranoid.

Organic brain damage is not confined to elderly patients. It may be present in chronic alcoholism, mental retardation, and head trauma, but the most common cause is cerebral arteriosclerosis and senile degeneration.

The behaviors displayed may differ depending upon which side of the brain is affected. Patients with left-side damage may have difficulty speaking and in understanding words. Patients with right-side damage may have difficulty with perceptual and spatial relationships - confuse up and down, right and left, walk into objects, have trouble following a straight line or dressing.

When the patient has trouble with language, he is helped and considered cooperative. When the patient cannot dress himself, follow directions, and continually bumps into things, he may be considered uncooperative or senile, a hopeless case.

OVERT BEHAVIOR

1. Memory loss for recent events, fair or good memory for past events, narrowing of interests, disorientation and confusion; fussy and exacting, he fights change and maintains rigid patterns of behavior, misplaces things, finds them, loses them again.
2. Reduced activity is nonproductive. He may be agitated or depressed, cheat or lie and be "mean" to others.
3. Bowel and bladder incontinence.
4. Sexual deviations (child molesting).
5. May react to illness with delirium.
6. Delirious, hallucinations, etc.

THE CONCEPT OF LONELINESS

The delusions and hallucinations of the aged can also be explained within the concept of loneliness. Loneliness is not the same as isolation, solitude or alienation. Loneliness is not the same as aloneness and distinction between the two is important when formulating intervention tactics. If a person feels aloneness, he withdraws voluntarily; if he feels loneliness, he is withdrawn involuntarily, feeling that he has been separated and isolated by external forces. In extreme loneliness there is the feeling that no human being in the world can ever relate to him. Aloneness can be constructive; loneliness is destructive. Lack of distinction between loneliness and aloneness motivates psychiatric nurses to foster "togetherness" in the therapeutic milieu, counterproductively insisting on continual interaction and participation. Denying the patient some time for aloneness prohibits him the opportunities for personal reintegration.

Existential psychoanalytic theorists have helped to delineate the two concepts of loneliness and aloneness. Sullivan believed components of loneliness begin in infancy and counteractions can be found in each developmental stage; the need for tenderness in infants, the expressive play of children, the juvenile peer group and the need for intimate relationships in adolescence.

In defining loneliness, Clark thought that man has a need to transcend his separateness which causes tension. Relief of his tension is sought through self-transcendence by direct (interpersonal relationships) or indirect (creative expression) means. If these means are successful, loneliness is relieved, at least temporarily. If these means are unsuccessful, barriers such as guilt, shame, self-alienation develop. If the barriers cannot be overcome, tension increases leading to increased anxiety and a greater degree of loneliness. Persistent unfulfilled needs lead to increased anxiety and psychic pain. To decrease anxiety and guard against pain such defenses as denial, suppression, repression, alcoholism and somatic complaints are used causing additional alienation and leading to more anxiety and loneliness. When the defensive measures no longer work, defenses may crumble and the lonely individual escapes to a world of unreality (personality disintegration).

PSYCHODYNAMICS

The psychodynamics of senility are not well understood. It is a life-long process and does not occur overnight. The organic and physio-logical changes in old age interact with the basic personality structure. Identical environmental stresses may provoke extreme reactions in one individual and be successfully coped with by another.

The personality is usually rigid and compulsive. He is a perfection-ist and has not learned to bend, so he breaks instead. The ego, which has controlled internal and external stimuli for years, cannot cope with the signs of physical deterioration, the knowledge that he is no longer useful, the thought that life is almost over.

He may regress to the oral stage and express some of his id im-pulses. He becomes childlike in his desire for love and affection, but maintains his adult desire for independence. He has problems once again with autonomy, and sometimes with basic trust.

He loses much of his ability to abstract; his thinking becomes more concrete and he is again egocentric. His thought processes inter-fere with his behaviors and sometimes dictate his behaviors.

His world becomes more narrow so that he can maintain control over it. Change and surprise may precipitate psychotic reactions as easily as loss and frustration.

Although there is no way back from senility, the regressive pattern may be halted and more appropriate behaviors substituted. He may continue with the developmental tasks of old age and continue to function.

NURSING INTERVENTIONS

1. Communication: Support and build up his feelings of self-worth. He wants most of all to be useful, accept him as he is - peevish, irritable, slow, forgetful; don't reject him in nonverbal behavior while accepting him verbally; any communication will be influ-enced by the symptoms displayed and will be different with a pa-tient displaying paranoid symptoms and one showing confusion, but it is usually easy to approach and establish a relationship with him.
2. Physical care:
   a. Diet. Simple meals; largest meal around the noon hour. Food should be easily digested, nutritious, and in small quantities. Unless otherwise indicated, he will need less meat and more milk and vegetables. He needs time to eat, attractive servings (his taste sense is dulled), and the chance to choose his own foods when he can. Absolutely necessary that his own teeth or dentures be well cared for and in a "use-ful" condition.
   b. Sleep. He may have trouble sleeping and doesn't need as much sleep. He does need rest, however. Needs to be kept as active as possible and discouraged from napping during the day if he will then be awake all night. A lack of privacy may

interfere with his sleeping if he shares a room. If old people are separated from their mates, they often cannot sleep.

Physical measures are helpful. Warm milk, back rubs, and just sitting with him may relax him and make him feel secure enough to sleep. Sometimes old people are afraid to fall asleep for fear they will not ever awaken. Just talking, sitting, and showing an interest may help.

c. Skin. Incontinence is dangerous for older, drier, less elastic skins. Needs to bathe less often in old age but needs to be "cleaned" whenever necessary. All soap should be removed from the skin, lotions applied, and any minor abrasions cared for immediately, because of poor circulation. The feet in particular, need attention.

d. Appearance. Failing eyesight and motor retardation may interfere with ability to dress appropriately. He may become fussy, take more time, be unable to decide what to wear. He may be incontinent and not change his clothes. He may refuse to change and insist upon wearing the same clothes every day - and sleeping in them at night. Needs encouragement to look his best, to get shaved, to wear his own clothes and to keep his clothes clean and cared for. Needs privacy when dressing.

3. Protection: He needs protection from himself. Suicide is common among the old, especially among men. He is also confused and may wander off. He may fall asleep smoking, or trip over objects too small for him to see. Constant observation is needed. He should not be out of sight for long periods of time. He may steal things and other patients need to be protected from his orneriness, stealing, and aggression. He also needs to be protected against further deterioration and loss of esteem. Reestablish bowel and bladder control when possible. Help him in making judgments to protect him from humiliation. Help him in his orientation - delusions are fixed but delirium and illusions can be explained. If illusions keep him awake, a night light may also help. His physical environment needs to be as safe as possible.

4. Recreation: Needs group activities that increase his feelings of belonging and his self-worth. Individual hobbies and activities are also therapeutic as long as they are not beyond his abilities. Activities need to be structured yet with some freedom of movement. Tasks requiring little time to be completed and not too much concentration can help rebuild his self-esteem.

The nurse's basic task with the senile patient is to provide him with a safe orderly environment, care for his physical needs, work with his strengths, protect him from himself and help resocialize him with group activities and hobbies.

REVIEW QUESTIONS

1. What are the main factors involved in the process of senility?
2. How can illusions be handled?
3. How does this differ from the approach to delusional behavior?
4. What is the most important need of the older patient?

5. What are some of the behaviors observable in the senile patient?
6. Does he need much physical care?
7. What does he need protection from the most?
8. What psychodynamics are involved in senility?
9. What developmental processes are involved?

SUGGESTED REFERENCES

1. Browne, L.J. and Ritter, J.I.: Reality therapy for the geriatric psychiatric patient, Perspectives Psychi Care X:135-139, 1972

2. Burnside, I.M.: Psychosocial Nursing; Care of the Aged, McGraw-Hill Book Co., New York, 1973

3. Clark, E.: Aspects of loneliness: Toward a framework of nursing intervention, In Developing Behavioral Concepts in Nursing, Southern Regional Educational Board, Georgia, pp. 35-50, 1968

4. Culbert, P. and Kos, B.: Aging: Considerations for health teaching, Nursing Clinics N Am, pp. 605-640, Dec., 1971

5. Ebersole, P.: Reminiscing, Am J Nursing, pp. 1304-1305, Aug., 1976

6. Ferraro, A.: Presenile psychoses, American Handbook of Psychiatry, Arieti, S., Ed., Basic Books, Inc., New York, Vol. II, pp. 1046-1077, 1959

7. Ferraro, A.: Senile psychoses, American Handbook of Psychiatry, Arieti, S., Ed., Basic Books, Inc., New York, Vol. II, pp. 1021-1045, 1959

8. Friedeman, J.S.: Cry for help: Suicide in the aged, J Gerontological Nursing II:28-32, May-June, 1976

9. Gresham, M.: The infantilization of the elderly: A developing concept, Nursing Forum XV:195-210, 1976

10. Hutchins, M.H.: The geriatric patient: Help me, Nursing Clinics N Am, pp. 795-805, Dec., 1971

11. Lehman, E.: Reality orientation, Nursing 1974 III:61-63, March, 1974

12. Maddox, G.L.: Disengagement theory: A critical evaluation, Gerontologist, pp. 80-83, April, 1964

13. Markson, J.: The timetable of old age, Am J Psychi, pp. 36-37, Feb., 1973

14. Moustakas, C.E.: Loneliness, Prentice-Hall, Inc., New York 1961

15. Peplau, H.: Loneliness, Am J Nursing LV:1476-1478, Dec., 1955

16. Preston, T.: When words fail, Am J Nursing, pp. 2064-2066, Dec., 1973

17. Roberts, J.: Loneliness, Perspectives Psychi Care X:226-231, 1972

18. Rynerson, B.: Need for self-esteem in the aged, A literature review, J Psychi Nursing Mental Health Nursing, pp. 22-26, Jan.-Feb., 1972

19. Sullivan, H.S.: Concepts of Modern Psychiatry, William Allison White Foundation, Washington, D.C., 1947

PART III: TREATMENT

CHAPTER 16

CHILD THERAPIES

PLAY ASSESSMENT AND THERAPY

Childhood has been described as a time of "trial run", when children
are given the play opportunities needed to find out about themselves
and the world in which they live. Play is a spontaneous, natural
form of self expression for the child, the child's self-initiated effort
to synthesize, adjust and control himself and his feelings. The
power of play for children is in its use for body, social and personality development, for learning and creativity.

Play provides the child a private reality of his own and protects his
egocentric world when he is forced to accommodate to everyday
living. Children play out anxieties, fears, anticipatory stress situations and curiosity. Since it is not possible to get a child to talk as
an adult, play is a natural way to have a child "act-out" what's going
on with him.

Play activity serves as a reassuring introduction between the child
and the nurse, a nondeceptive encounter which relieves tensions.
Play can be used as indirect preparation for uncomfortable or "unusual" examinations and procedures. For example, the following
play and games can be used by the nurse in a simple neurological
evaluation of a child:

1. Cerebral Functions: "Hide and Seek"; "Let's copy these drawings"; "Simon Says"; "Blindman's Bluff"; "Naming Games".
2. Reflexes: "Let's Tell Our Bodies To --"; "Let's Take Turns";
   "You Play Nurse".
3. Cerebellar Functions: "Follow the Leader"; "Patty Cake"; "Pin
   the Tail on the Donkey"; and imitative gymnastics as: "Make a
   Fist"; "Ring Around the Rosey"; and "Indian Wrestling".
4. Sensory Functions: "Hot and Cold"; "Tickling Games"; "Body
   Tapping Games"; and "Touching Games".
5. Cranial Nerves: "Play Dentist"; "Smelling Games"; "Following
   Lights"; and "Whispering Games" (Duffy).

By watching a child at play, much can be learned about his real
and imaginary emotional life. If a playroom or private hospital
area is used, sex and age appropriate toys and play material
should be assembled prior to the assessment. Diagnostic play assessments are unstructured play observations made with a therapist
"set" of attitudes through which the child can feel free to express
himself. While assessment is ongoing and adapted to the changing
behaviors of the child, the initial play assessment provides a baseline for future play therapy or the decision for alternate forms of
therapy. The initial play assessment, like the adult's mental status
examination, focuses on diagnostic clues and takes between 30 to 45

minutes. The nurse therapist acts as a participant observer as she completes some of the following tasks:

1. Establishing a climate of trust and understanding.
2. Providing play mediums through which the child can express himself.
3. Learning the child's vocabulary, i.e., the names he uses for persons, places, and objects.

Some of the things to be learned from a diagnostic play session are:

1. The child's internal fears, concerns, and apprehensions.
2. How the child sees the world and tests reality.
3. The child's general mood and affective capacity.
4. How the child relates to adults other than his parents.
5. The child's ego defenses.
6. The child's ability for mastery and learning.
7. The child's mobility, coordination and frustration tolerance
8. The child's manner of relating.
9. Gender configuration.
10. Developmental level.
11. The child's concept of his problems.
12. The child's attention span.

The anxious child may be so inhibited he cannot play; the hyperactive child may handle all the play materials quickly, starting every game available but completing none. Some children compulsively line toys in careful order while others aggressively toss them about. Some cautiously and delicately touch play materials; others angrily grasp. Some avoid clay and "messy" things while others delight in smearing. Often a stressed child reverts to earlier developmental periods, choosing highly charged symbolic materials and playing with them in a regressive manner, as the 10-year-old that sucks the baby dolls' bottle and babbles.

After assessment, the decision for type of treatment evolves from evaluation of the family as well as the child's problems. Treatment of the child may be by individual treatment of the child or mother, couple therapy with parenting guidance, conjoint family, sibling, dyad (child and parent) group, or filial therapy (parents learning to be the therapeutic agents).

In sophisticated psychiatric in-patient settings, evaluation of a child includes interdisciplinary team evaluations as psychological tests (CAT), tests for I.Q. (usually WISC), learning styles, cognitive capacity, perceptual motor functioning, and projective tests as Draw A Person. Family interviews and naturistic observations of the child at home, in school and at play provide additional information to understanding the child and his social system.

PLAY THERAPY

Play therapy is a professional method of using play with nonthreatening attitudes and play materials to discover and resolve what is troubling a child. Play is the child's language, the toys and materials are the child's words. Play therapy techniques have been described and delineated as follows:

1. Play analysis: Direct and verbal interpretations made of the child's behavior during play, to gain access to the child's most deeply and repressed feelings and fixations.
2. Structured (directive) play therapy: The introduction of specific procedures to achieve a goal. Frequently used in "anticipatory" play therapy prior to traumatic hospital procedures and with mentally retarded and/or organically impaired children. The therapeutic use of play to develop child's ability to learn, experience, and broaden his understanding of his life experience.
3. Unstructured (nondirective) play therapy: The child's use of toys in fantasy play to express conflict symbolically and to reduce anxiety by restructuring his life in a play situation he can control.

Anna Freud was the first to use play therapy with children, noting that the daydreams of children and the activity of their fantasy equals the free association of adults in analysis. Fantasy is the name given to daydreaming as opposed to controlled thought. Play therapy is the system of child analysis best suited for neurotic behavior problems by investigating the child's ego.

Children create a world of fantasy for themselves in play. The denial of reality is a feature of child's play in general, but especially in their games of make believe. The healthy child can grasp the difference between fantasy and reality and gets involved in explorations of the real world; the disturbed child cannot make this transition. The task of play therapy is to get the child to separate fantasy and fact and to help him assimilate reality into his world and the general scheme of things. The therapist assists with the process by gradually understanding the illogical manifestations of the child's play and by providing a corrective environment for him to "play them through".

Play therapy is most useful for children between the ages of three and twelve. Since the child has difficulty in verbalizing his feelings, dramatic play is encouraged by the use of mutual storytelling, puppet play for role modeling and unstructured materials as clay, crayons, and finger paints.

Imaginative doll play is a "natural mode" for little girls, while G. I. Joes and other male dolls now available provide excellent, socially acceptable doll play for little boys. Dolls are often given names by the child of significant others in the child's life and one doll may become the child's own projected self. Stressful past and present anticipated threatening situations are played out and often the child asks the therapist to actively take a "doll's role". This provides a vehicle for the therapist's reflections of the child's feelings. In this technique, the therapist repeats without interpretation what the child is expressing to:

1. Indicate the therapist's empathy
2. Clarify the child's feelings
3. Provide the child opportunity for insight

The child's diffused and undifferentiated emotions and feelings presented when play therapy begins become focused to specific situations, are dealt with ambivalently and finally resolved in a positive manner. Often children "terminate" their own therapy sessions, identifying they no longer "need to play about that" nor require additional therapeutic encounters. For the child to learn to use the play medium therapeutically, to grasp what is no longer "felt" or needed to be played out with the supportive adult, careful "structuring" of the therapy sessions is essential.

The "structuring" or building the relationship so the child understands the therapy process and is able to use the sessions meaningfully is the cornerstone to effective play therapy. Axline (pp. 73-74) lists eight basic principles for structuring nondirective play therapy contacts to assure proper structure. These direct the therapist by:

1. Developing a warm, friendly relationship with the child.
2. Accepting the child exactly as he is.
3. Establishing a feeling of permissiveness so child feels free to express his feelings.
4. Being alert to the feelings the child expresses and reflecting them back to the child so he can gain insight into his behavior.
5. Respecting the child's ability to solve his own problems and supporting the child's choice toward making changes.
6. Allowing the child, not the therapist, to lead the way (initiate conversation, etc.).
7. Not hurrying the process.
8. Setting needed limits, indicating to the child the therapist's responsibility in the relationship.

A concept of "normal" play activities also provides the therapist a conceptual framework for age, central themes, fantasies, play materials and secondary gains (Allen). Briefly, these activities are:

Group I: Central theme of anxieties concerning the body. Feelings of helplessness may be denied by compensatory fantasies of grandeur. Play materials preferred are those related to body functions and body parts.

Group II: Central theme relating to preoedipal mother relationships and the fear of loss of love objects. Repetition, mirroring play, using maternal play with dolls and stuffed animals. Play focuses on learning to delay gratification.

Group III: Oedipal relations and defenses against them begin about three years of age. Spontaneous doll and dramatic play occurs with a wide variety of emotions, roles, and plots with fantasies of a social, creative nature. Co-play is common, by which the child prepares for adult roles.

Group IV: Sibling relations and fear of the superego, start about six years of age. The importance of rules, codes, rituals through board games as chess and checkers are common. Organized co-play to learn cooperation with siblings, peers, and parents predominate.

Play therapy with psychotic children (Ekstein) differs from the therapeutic approach used with neurotic and emotionally disturbed children. Psychotic children vacillate between symbiotic and autistic states and are usually in primary process, the creative, imaginary "reverie" period during which time and space have no impact. The therapeutic intervention with psychotic children is to use the metaphor through which child makes contact with the outer world. Interpretation of behavior may increase the psychotic child's need to retreat to his inner world of sameness.

PLAY GROUPS

Play therapy groups of five or six children are useful for children with emotional problems as: impulse control, expressions of aggression, autonomy, regressive behaviors, inconsistent parenting, sibling rivalry and developmental issues. The decision for a heterogenous or homogenous group depends on the developmental task in progress; however, it is usually unwise to assemble a group of children with the same problem (as regressive or aggressive behaviors). By using group processes, the child's peer interactions are used in the corrective process. Play groups also help the members to:

1. Develop more positive self-concepts.
2. Increase their frustration tolerance.
3. Delay gratification.
4. Verbalize rather than act-out feelings.
5. Develop acceptable outlets for aggression expression.
6. Become comfortable in the structure of a group.
7. Improve peer relationships.

The group members provide the child "models" and alternatives to his present behavior repertoire. The therapist may identify a child's behavior to the other children, asking their suggestions for "better" ways of problem solving. Thus, the group grows and shares its past learnings; the group also provides the child the opportunity to apply new learnings in a peer interaction setting and have guidance during the accommodation process.

PLAY THERAPY AND THE CHILD HOSPITALIZED FOR MEDICAL-SURGICAL PROBLEMS

Hospitalization causes radical changes in the child's life, presenting potential sources of neurotic anxiety as fear of the loss of love and the risk of injury and pain at the hands of others. Anna Freud was among the first authority to observe that physical illness in children could precipitate neurotic disturbances in childhood and adult life; Morrissey's later research with dying children statistically verified Freuds' observation. He found most of the children had considerable anxiety about hospitalization and expressed this concern verbally, behaviorally, symbolically and physiologically. His recommendations were that hospitalized children have direct therapeutic services for these emotional needs as a routine part of medical-surgical hospitalization to prevent future emotional problems.

While the research and literature on play therapy documents its critical synthesizing role in the mental health of children, medical-surgical nurses have been slow in implementing the healing power of play in their pediatric interventions. The children's intense requirements for physical attention in most pediatric units limits the pediatric nurse's time and opportunity for implementing play intervention.

Despite these time constraints, however, a growing number of articles describing ego-oriented programs for pediatric clients to re-enact, face and master the hospital experience, have recently appeared in the nursing literature. Play is also being used in anticipatory guidance prior to intrusive and traumatic procedures. While miniature hospitals, syringes and "nurse and doctor dolls" provide elaborate stimuli for play therapy on the pediatric unit, a few simple toys, props and an attentive adult is often all that is required to alleviate the hospitalized child's stress.

Most children requiring hospitalization fear separation, mutilation and death. The child's focus of anxiety varies with maturation levels: the young child is most concerned about his physical security, comfort and maternal separation; the preschooler is concerned with his autonomy, shame and bodily invasion. The schoolage child is most concerned with losing his sense of mastery, control and independence.

Grief commonly occurs in children with chronic illnesses that involve changes in their body image, physical freedom and their anticipated normal growth and development. Grief can often best be resolved through nondirective play. The three phases of childhood grief are (Bowlby):

1. Protest and denial
2. Pain, despair and disorganization
3. Hope and adaptation

Any situation in which the child's resistance to frustration is lowered raises the child's stress level and threatens his immature ego apparatus. Many hospitalized children become more aggressive when they are thwarted in their need for physical activity by confinement to a bed or hospital unit. The dramatic play which involves physical violence and the use of aggression in fantasy frequently seen in the hospitalized child does not always correspond to the child's real life. Such play is often the child's attempts to handle aggressive impulses with primitive defenses of projection and fantasy.

The Hospital Picture Test (Barton, 1964) is a useful projective test that helps identify areas of the child's fantasy-stress and provides prescriptive direction to the emotional areas needing play therapy intervention.

PREVENTATIVE PLAY TECHNIQUES

Principles of play therapy have been adapted to schools and class-rooms and the use of parents and teachers as therapists has recently been explored. The Human Classroom (Moustakas) emphasizes play as the vehicle for learning and self-actualizing of the normal child.

Brody has evolved a concept of "developmental play", which is based on Bowlby's attachment theories. Through physical activities and body contact, the child and a significant adult develop an attachment relationship, which is the basis for cognitive, social and emotional growth. The "sculpting" of relationships with well children provides the nurse an initial experience for developing the skills of play inter-action essential to the concepts of play therapy, as well as opportunity to integrate physical, emotional, cognitive and social develop-mental theories.

BEHAVIOR THERAPIES

Behavior therapies and behavior modification are terms used inter-changeably to describe attempts to change behavior using learning theory. Psychologists believe that behavior is learned and behavior that has been learned can be unlearned by "reconditioning". The proponents of behavior therapy claim it is a superior form of treat-ment because it has a scientific, theoretical base that requires ob-jective analysis, description and quantification of a clinical problem. Psychologists use more behavior therapy than any other form of treatment and there are more publications on behavior therapy in the psychology literature than on any other form of treatment. While behavior therapies are also used with adults, their widespread use by teachers and therapists working with children and with parents as in Parent Effectiveness Training (PET) make behavior therapies one of the most popular and widely used techniques currently em-ployed in changing children's maladaptive behaviors.

Behavior therapies use conditioning principles, in contrast to the principles of the psychoanalytic process of insight into the uncons-cious. In the behavioral therapies, the patient does not "work through" his problem. "Working through", is the process by which a patient discovers, piece by piece, over periods of time, the impli-cations of an insight or interpretation and gradually comes to under-stand the implications of that insight on one's behavior. The process of "working through" and "conditioning" principles are basic to the differ-ences of the two therapeutic approaches. Instead of focusing on intrapsychic abnormalities as excessive anxieties, poor impulse control and character defects, behavior therapies focus on patterns of response in the social environment. The patient, child or parent actively participates in the therapy and has a clear idea of what be-havior he is to change, and what will happen as a direct consequence of the behavioral manifestation.

Behavior therapies use learning theory, which focus on the connec-tion between environmental stimuli and a person's behavior response (S-R bond). Two models are derived from the S-R bond of learning theory:

1. Classical conditioning: Pavlovian theory, in which a stimulus elicits a response, as the sight of food (stimulus), causes salivation (response).
2. Operant conditioning: Skinnerian theory, which claims a response is more likely to occur if it is reinforced than a response that is not reinforced.

The consequences of behavior, the positive or negative reinforcement, determine the frequency of a response. Positive reinforcements are consequences that increase the likelihood of a response occurring again; punishment or aversion (negative reinforcement) decrease the possibility of the event occurring again. Reinforcers or "tokens" can be primary, as food and substances (usually raisins and milk with children) rewarding basic primary needs. Secondary reinforcers are usually social approval or disapproval and social privileges, as participation in social activities.

Overcoming habitual, repetitive maladaptive behavior also involves modeling and shaping. By "shaping" a therapist reinforces successive approximations until the desired behavior is achieved. "Successive approximations" refers to a step-by-step process in which the child is moved toward a desired goal. In order to develop a successful shaping program, the desired behavior must already exist in the child's behavioral repertoire - if it does not exist, the reinforcer can inadvertently reinforce behavior that is undesirable. Children learn to speak by "successive approximations", and shaping protocols have been successfully used with children who are electively mute, stutter, are ecolalic, or have other verbal/vocal communication problems.

By "modeling" the therapist demonstrates the desired behavior, teaching by demonstration the behaviors the patient does not have in his behavioral repertoire. Many behavior modification programs require "modeling" before shaping can be established. Bandura lists three major effects of modeling behavior on the observer (child):

1. The observer may acquire new patterns of behavior that did not previously exist in his behavioral repertoire. Novel behaviors modeled are quickly reproduced by the observer with almost identical imitation. Children are especially quick to imitate and learn by observing others.
2. Modeling weakens or strengthens the observer's behavior if he sees that behavior rewarded or punished. This is especially true if the child has a relationship or "identity" with the person modeling.
3. Modeling behaviors are generalized to other areas as the observer integrates them into their repertoire. For example, the child who has learned to put things away after a play therapy session with the therapist will often pick up his toys at home after play.

To establish a behavior therapy program, initial baseline and ongoing assessments are essential. Initial baseline assessment includes:

1. The determination of the behavior to be changed.
2. The frequency the behavior occurs (how often?)
3. The situations in which the undesirable behavior occurs; where, when, and under what conditions the behavior will or will not occur.
4. The reinforcers that appear to be responsible for the child to continue his maladaptive behavior.

Adequate records on the frequency of the behavior occurring confirms a behavioral diagnosis. Frequency charts and the continued tallying of behavioral occurrences during the treatment provides numerical evidence of the success or failure of the behavior modification program.

Protocols of behavioral response programs are carefully specified so that the staff members, the child's family, or teachers consistently reinforce the same behavior with the same reinforcers.

With emotionally disturbed children, positive primary reinforcers are generally most effective since often the child has poor relationships with adults and does not respond to "social" rewards. For example, a child is taught to dress (before breakfast, using the child's natural hunger state) by giving him an M and M or raisin each time he makes the correct step in the dressing procedure. Incorrect steps are ignored since he is more inclined to do those things for which he is rewarded, the desired behavior is programmed.

Bio-feedback, instructions, behavioral rehearsal, assertive training, and behavioral contracting are forms of behavioral therapies currently in use. The most important consideration in planning any behavioral therapy project is the selection of a reward which is "rewarding" to the unique personality of the child and to select a step sequence that is challenging. Assurance of consistent environmental responses is also important; unless all persons in contact with the child's behavior participate in the program, it is unlikely it will succeed. For example, to alter a child's compulsive swearing, teachers, parents and peers must all participate in the behavior modification program for it to be effective. The environmental responders must be consistent in the reinforcements.

The introduction of behavioral modification techniques in psychiatric settings has added depth and precision to psychiatric nurses' observation of patient behaviors as well as improved collaboration between nursing team members. Specific behavior scales describing aspects of patient behaviors have been organized by psychologists and these scales are widely used by the nursing staffs to identify subtle changes in patient behavior. The Nursing Observation Scale for Inpatient Evaluation (NOSIE) is an example of a behavioral scale formulated by psychologists and useful for evaluating subtle behavioral changes in response to medication, sleep patterns and environmental manipulation. The scales are specific and unambiguous; nurses, aides, and other staff can evaluate and make description of the patient's behavior in a consistent form.

Behavior modification has been reported successful in the treatment of enuresis, encorporesis, temper tantrums, school phobias, anorexia nervosa, obsessions, and the correction of many maladaptive behaviors and neurotic problems. Critics of behavior modification techniques caution that (Shapiro):

1. Alleviation of one symptom may precipitate other, more serious maladaptive behaviors.
2. Caution should be used in focusing on a symptom that is organically caused and cannot be unlearned and might better be treated by medication.
3. The complexities and interweaving of psychiatric symptomology should not be overlooked by focusing on a specific behavior.

No matter what form of treatment is used in intervening with behavioral and emotional disturbances of childhood, the younger the child, the more quickly positive results are usually achieved. Young children tend to respond more quickly to treatment than adolescents or adults because:

1. They are naturally curious, imitative and intervention efforts flow into their normal "growing and learning process".
2. Ego defenses are recently acquired in the child's immature personality structure and these defenses are more fluid and less fixed than in older persons.

"Brief" therapy refers to intervention of less than six months' time duration, and usually 12 to 15 play or psychotherapeutic sessions are sufficient when intervening with children's emotional problems. When specific time programs for behavior modification are established - as "morning dressing behavior protocols" - 12 to 15 20-minute sessions are generally the maximum number of sessions; if no behavior changes occur, reassessment and implementation of other approaches are indicated.

REVIEW QUESTIONS

1. Why is play used to assess children?
2. How do play therapy and play assessment differ?
3. What are the indications for using behavior modification?
4. What are the steps in behavior modification?
5. How do play therapy and behavior modification differ?
6. When would you use play therapy instead of behavior modification?

SUGGESTED REFERENCES

1. Ables, E.S. and Aug, R.G.: Pitfalls encountered by beginning child therapist, Psychotherapy: Theory, Research and Practice, pp. 9-14, Winter, 1972

2. Adams, M.: A hospital play program: Helping children with serious illness, Am J Orthopsychi XLVI:416-424, July, 1976

3. Adams, P.L.: A Primer of Child Psychiatry, Little, Brown & Co., Boston, 1974

4. Allen, F.: Therapy as a living experience, In Psychotherapy with Children, Moustakas, C., Ed., Ballantine Books, New York, 1970

5. Axline, V.: Play Therapy, Ballantine Books, New York, 1947

6. Bandura, A.: Psychotherapy based upon modeling procedures, Handbook of Psychotherapy and Behavior Change, Bergin, A.E. and Garfield, S.L., Eds., John Wiley & Sons, New York, pp. 653-708, 1971

7. Barbero, G.J.: Cyclic vomiting, Pediatrics, pp. 740-746, 1960

8. Barnard, K.E. and Erickson, M.L.: Teaching Children with Developmental Problems, 2nd Ed., C.V. Mosby, New York, 1976

9. Barnard, M.U. and Wolf, L.: Psychosocial failure to thrive: Nursing assessment and intervention, Nursing Clinics N Am III:557-565, Sept., 1973

10. Barton, P.: Nursing assessment and intervention through play, Current Issues in Psychotherapy, Carsinni, R., Ed., Harper & Row, New York, pp. 203-217, 1968

11. Barton, P.: The Relationship Between Overt and Fantasy Stress Reactions of Children to Hospitalization, Doctoral dissertation, University of Florida, Gainesville, Fla., 1964

12. Berlin, J.N.: Advocacy for Children's Mental Health, Brunner-Mazel, New York, 1976

13. Berni, E. and Fordyce: Behavior Modification and the Nursing Process, C.V. Mosby, St. Louis, 1973

14. Blyth, Z.: Group treatment for handicapped children, J Psychi Nursing Mental Health Services VII:172-176, July-Aug., 1969

15. Bowlby, J.: Attachment and Loss: Vol. I; Attachment: Vol. II; Anxiety and Anger, Basic Books, New York, 1969

16. Braff, D.L.: Clinical and theoretical consequences of misuse of basis behavior therapy concept, Am J Psychi CXXX:820-821, 1973

17. Brazelton, T.B.: Infants and Mothers: Differences in Development, Delacorte Press, New York, 1970

18. Brody, V.: Sourcebook for Finding Your Way to Helping Young Children Through Developmental Play, Pupil Personnel Services Demonstration Project, All Childrens Hospital, St. Petersburg, Fla., State of Florida, 1976

19. Browning, R.M.: Behavior Modification in Child Treatment, Aldine-Atherton Press, Chicago, 1971

20. Caplan, F. and Caplan, T.: The Power of Play, Doubleday Anchor Books, New York, 1973

21. Carigan, T.: Self-motivation and self-control in operant conditioning, Perspectives Psychi Care XII:96-104, 1974

22. Casolyn, T.: Affective development in psychotic boy, Perspectives Psychi Care IX:34-39, 1971

23. Clements, P.: Teaching children to be their own behavior therapist, J School Health, 1973

24. Duffy, J.C.: Child Psychiatry, Medical Examination Publishing Co., New York, 1974

25. Erickson, E.H.: Play and actuality, Play and Development, Piers, M., Ed., W.W. Norton, New York, 1972

26. Freud, S.: Little Hans, The Sexual Enlightenment of Children, Collier Books, New York, 1963

27. Freud, A.: The role of bodily illness in the mental life of the child, Psychoanalytic Study Child VII:69-81, 1952

28. Gardner, R.: Mutual Story-Telling as a Technique in Child Psychotherapy: Science and Psychoanalysis XIV:123-136, 1969

29. Geiser, R.L. and Norberta, S.M.: Sexual disturbance in young children, Maternal Child Nursing, pp. 187-194, May-June, 1976

30. Gesell, A., et al.: Infant and Child in the Culture Today, Harper & Row, New York, 1974

31. Ginott, H.: Play group therapy: A theoretical framework, International J Group Psychother VIII:410-413, 1958

32. Ginsberg, B.G.: Parents as therapeutic agents: The usefulness of filial therapy in a community mental health center, Am J Community Psychol VI:47-54, March, 1976

33. Goldstein, A.: Behavior Therapy: Current Psychotherapies, Corsini, R., Ed., Peacock Publishers, Itasca, Ill., 1973

34. Goodman, J.D. and Sours, J.A.: The Child Mental Status Examination, Basic Books, Inc., New York, 1967

35. Grollman, E.A., Ed.: Explaining Death to Children, Beacon Press, Boston, 1967

36. Hartley, R.E., et al.: Understanding Children's Play, Columbia University Press, New York, 1952

37. Henry, J.: Pathways to Madness, Random House, New York, 1965

38. Jenkins, R.L.: The runaway reaction, Am J Psychi CXXVIII: 168-173, 1971

39. Kestenberg, J., et al.: Development of the young child as expressed through bodily movement, J Am Psychoanalytic Assoc XIX:746-764, 1971

40. Kestenberg, J.: How children remember and parents forget, International J Psychoanalytic Psychother II:103-123, May, 1972

41. Koppitz, E.M.: Psychological Evaluation of Children's Human Figure Drawings, Grune & Stratton, New York, 1968

42. Lanchester, J.: Activity groups as therapy, Am J Nursing LXXVI:948-949, June, 1976

43. Lazarus, A.A. and Abramowitz, A.: The use of "emotive imagery" in the treatment of children's phobias, J Mental Sci CVIII:191-195, 1962

44. LeCompte, W.F., et al.: Effects of training on behavioral observations by nurses, Nursing Research XXI:448-452, Sept.-Oct., 1972

45. Loveffelt, M.: Play in Childhood, John Wiley & Sons, New York, 1967

46. Mann, J.: Time Limited Psychotherapy, The Harvard University Press, Cambridge, Mass., 1973

47. Morrison, T.L. and Newcomer, B.: Effects of directive versus nondirective play therapy with institutionalized mentally retarded children, Am J Mental Deficiency CXXIX:666-669, 1975

48. Morrissey, J.: Children's adaptation to fatal illness, Social Work VIII:81-88, 1963

49. Moustakas, C.E. and Cereta, P.: Learning to be Free, Prentice Hall, New Jersey, 1973

50. Moustakas, C.E., Ed., Psychotherapy with Children: The Living Relationship, Ballantine Books, New York, 1959

51. Moustakas, C.E.: Who Will Listen? Children and Parents in Therapy, Ballantine Books, New York, 1975

52. Mundy, J.: The use of projective techniques with children, Manual of Child Psychopathology, Wolman, B., Ed., McGraw Hill, New York, 1972

53. Ohlson, E.L.: The meaningfulness of play for children and parents: An effective counseling strategy, J Family Counseling XI:53-54, Spring, 1974

54. Petrillo, M. and Sanger, S.: Emotional Care of the Hospitalized Child, Lippincott, Philadelphia, 1972

55. Poznanski, E.O., et al.: Childhood repression, J Acad Child Psychi XV:491-501, Summer, 1976

56. Rosecrans, C.J.: Play - The language of children, Mental Hygiene LIII:367-384, July, 1968

57. Rosenhan, D.L.: On being sane in insane places, Science CLXI: 250-258, Jan., 1973

58. Rosenthal, R. and Jackson, L.: Pygmalion in the Classroom, Holt, Rinehart & Co., New York, 1968

59. Ryleick, L.: Preparing parents to teach their children about human sexuality, Maternal Child Nursing III:182-185, May-June, 1974

60. Sands, R.M. and Gobele, S.: Breaking the bonds of tradition: A reassessment of group treatment of latency-age children, Am J Psychi CXXXI:662-665, June, 1974

61. Schapler, E.: Developmental Therapy for Autistic Children: Individual and Social Implications, Paper presented to the National Society for Autistic Children, Philadelphia, Pa., June, 1971

62. Shapiro, A.: The behavior therapies: Therapeutic breakthrough or latest fad? Am J Psychi CXXXIII:154-159, Feb., 1976

63. Slanson, S.R. and Schiffer, M.: Group Psychotherapies for Children: A Textbook, International Universities Press, New York, 1975

64. Task Force Report 5: Behavior Therapy in Psychiatry, American Psychiatric Association, Washington, D.C., 1973

65. Visintainer, M. and Wolfer, J.A.: Psychological preparation for surgical pediatric patients: The effects on children's and parents' stress responses and adjustment, Pediatrics CLVI: 187-202, Aug., 1975

66. Visotsky, H.: The joint commission on mental health of children: Progress report, Psychiatric Annals: The Mental Health of Children, pp. 213-220, June, 1975

67. Weinberger, G.: Brief therapy with children and their parents, In Barten, Ed., Brief Therapies, Behavioral Publications, New York, 1971

68. White, J.H., et al.: Treating infantile autism with parent therapist, International J Child Psychother I:83-95, 1972

CHAPTER 17

RELATIONSHIP THERAPIES

MARITAL THERAPY

Research findings indicate the two major reasons people seek psychiatric help are for marital and family problems (Berman and Lief). Despite the significance of family problems, the traditional emphasis on individual intrapsychic factors, the one-to-one relationship and fear of dilution of transference in joint therapy have slowed wide spread acceptance of marital therapy as a therapeutic technique. Marital counseling, with its broad anticipatory emphasis, differs from marital therapy, which uses unconscious factors and deals with transactional psychopathology. Confusion between, and misuse of the two terms and approaches has also hindered acceptance of marital and family therapy as legitimate psychotherapeutic methods.

Conceptual schemes of dyadic relationships include the three issues that all interactions must come to terms with:

1. How we communicate (the rules of formal aspects of communication from systems and communication theory).
2. What we communicate (the role expectations and behaviors from social psychology).
3. Why we communicate (the motivational explanations drawn from psychoanalytic concepts of early childhood experiences).

Marital relationships are classified according to four critical dimensions:

1. Power: Who's in charge? There are symmetrical, complimentary or parallel distributions of power.
2. Level of intimacy: What are the territorial imperatives of the couple? These are described as conflict-habituated, devitalized, passive-congenial, vital and total types of intimate relationships.
3. Psychodynamic levels: How do the individual character traits conflict or support the relationship in a "neurotic balance"? Utilizing the unconscious factors and needs that frequently attract couples to one another and the repetitious behaviors needed to carry psychic functions for each other, the dyads include: obsessive-compulsive husband - hysterical wife; passive dependent husband - dominant wife; paranoid husband - depressive prone wife; depressive husband - paranoid wife; and oral-dependent dyads such as neurotic wife and impotent husband.
4. Inclusion-exclusion: Who's included or excluded from the relationship? These are described as: before child rearing, early child rearing, latency and adolescent children and after the children leave.

The inclusion-exclusion dimensions evolve from a combining of adult developmental and marital tasks. Building on Erikson's theories of psychosocial development, adult developmental tasks and stages as they relate to the marital life cycle have been identified as follows (Berman and Lief):

Stage 1 (18-21 years): Pulling up roots and developing autonomy. The marital task is shifting from family to new commitment; the area of marital conflict is with original family ties. A fragile intimacy and testing of power and conflicts over in-laws threaten the marital boundaries during this stage.

Stage 2 (22-28 years): Provisional adulthood, a period of developing intimacy and occupational identification, with the task of provisional marital commitment. Marital conflicts are stresses over parenthood and uncertainty about choice of marital partner. Intimacy is deepening but ambivalent and patterns of conflict resolution over power issues are established. Work, friends and potential lovers challenge the marital boundaries.

Stage 3 (29-31 years): The transition at age 30 is characterized by restlessness, conflicts about work versus marriage, parenthood and increasing distance with partner while re-evaluation pervades. As the partners vie for power and dominance, there is a compensatory "fortress building" or extra-marital involvement.

Stage 4 (32-39 years): Period of settling down with deepening commitments and establishment of long range goals. Conflicts about ways productivity is achieved by partners, marked by a delineation of a "good" or "bad" marriage. The nuclear family closes its boundaries as dominance and decision-making patterns and powers are firmly established.

Stage 5 (40-42 years): Mid-life transition during which the individual searches for a "fit" between aspirations and reality, a summing up of the past and establishing new future goals. There are conflicts of individual success versus staying in the marriage, with increased fantasies about other relationships disrupting restabilization.

Stage 6 (43-59 years): Middle adulthood, usually characterized by restabilization and reordering of priorities, conflict resolution and "settling in". Concerns about losing youthfulness causes depression, acting-out and re-enactments of the Oedipal problem (if unresolved). The "empty nest syndrome" appears as children leave and intimacy between partners increases or decreases. Boundaries are fixed.

Stage 7 (60 and over): Older age requires the effective dealing with aging, illness and death. Marital conflicts and fears center on loneliness and sexual failure. There is a stable plateau of intimacy and marital boundaries solidify. The physical environment is critical in maintaining ties with the outside world for the aging couple.

The methods of marital therapy include the application of a variety of therapeutic tactics focusing on the transactional aspects of the marriage. Insight, behavior modification, role playing, group and individual dynamics provide the framework for these interventions. In marital therapy, the goal is not to restructure personality, but to help couples become more comfortable with their own dynamics and more flexible and open. The techniques used are:

Collaborative techniques: one-to-one treatment of the spouses by different therapists. This approach is best when spouses have widely different goals.

Concurrent techniques: both spouses are seen on a one-to-one basis by the same therapist; useful when both spouses have internal conflicts in addition to their marital problems and little insight into the contribution of their behavior to the marital discord.

Combined techniques: includes all available family members.

Conjoint techniques: the couple is seen by a therapist and/or co-therapist, and "therapeutic impasses" are dealt with in individual therapies. This triadic approach is best for marital disharmony, when there is a need to improve the communication process between spouses, and when marital problems have reached crisis proportions.

Five transference relationships in marital therapy have been identified (Green, 1970):

1. Transference to the therapist as a new person or new transactional encounter.
2. Transference symbolically represented within the context of the client's fantasy system.
3. Regressive transferences as in one-to-one relationships.
4. Triadic relationships may stimulate the Oedipal family triangle with competitive sibling and parental sentiments.
5. Adaptive feedback, the return of positive feelings to therapist and spouse, is facilitated.

Techniques and approaches of the therapist involve:

1. Focusing on current issues between the couple that are causing the conflict.
2. Facilitating and fostering alternate communication patterns.
3. Facilitating the expression of conflicts, acting as go-between, judiciously shifting sides to balance the relationship.
4. Utilizing psychodynamics in the positive interpretation of destructive behaviors.
5. Confronting couples on the relationships of past experiences in current reactions.
6. Maintaining positive feelings between marriage partners during and about destructive behaviors.

If marital therapy proceeds to family therapy (as when marital conflicts prohibit partners relating to the children), the parents will require assistance in shifting transference bonds established in the triadic situation.

FAMILY THERAPY

Family therapy uses naturally occurring, pre-established social units and introduces change in an on-going system. The main difference between individual and family therapy is the shift of focus from the sick person to the family's emotional process that created an "identified patient". Most of the theories and practice of family therapy have grown during the last two decades, a time when one out of five marriages fail and "zero" population growth is a goal.

A variety of schools of family therapy have developed techniques and theories reflecting the interdisciplinary use of the family as a unit of treatment. Marriage counselors, social workers, psychologists, sociologists and anthropologists provide therapeutic variations which span the spectrum from the analyst's couch to the group circle. The conceptual frameworks used in family study include: interactional, structure-functional, situational, institutional and developmental (Hill and Hansen). However, most of the evidence supports family therapy as beginning within psychiatry, an outgrowth of psychoanalytic technique. One of the earliest uses of family therapy was by Freud in his classical case of Little Hans.

Yet family therapy is a radical shift from the traditional psychoanalytic avoidance of interactions with the family that keeps the therapeutic relationship with the "identified" patient "uncontaminated".

While family therapy may be seen as another form of treatment for disturbed children, it varies from the classical child guidance model which assigns different therapists to parents and children. The therapist's role in family therapy is one of "involved impartiality" in which attention is focused on a set of relationships and individual advocacy becomes the contaminating factor. Family therapy is not just a new treatment method but a new way of conceptualizing the cause and cure of mental illness. A common assumption of family therapists is that, if a person is to change, the context in which he lives must change. The question is not "who" is the problem, but "what" is the trouble.

Treatment of the family unit is not group therapy. Families have a history prior to therapeutic intervention. They are ongoing systems with continued contacts from session to session; they have transferences, alliances and splits that they bring to the treatment situation. While group therapies aid in socialization and individual therapy removes autistic elements in an individual's pathology, family therapy changes on-going interaction patterns.

Treatment decisions: The diagnostic formulation underlying the selection of family therapy for treatment hinge on careful assessment of the meaning of the symptoms to the family, the communication patterns, the focus of the distress and the workable areas. While analysis of these areas depends in part on the therapist's frame of reference, some indications for family therapy are when:

1. The family constellation is available.
2. There are adolescent separation problems.

3. There is a trading of dissociations.
4. There is distancing.
5. There is cognitive chaos.

Contraindications for family therapy are:

1. When anxious, young parents are on the verge of decompensating or have recently recompensated from an acute psychotic breakdown.
2. When couples can't work out their own problems and be free enough to relate to children.
3. When family therapy is used to avoid change.

The treatment unit: While most family therapist's believe all persons who are involved in the family transactional system should be included in the family assessment, there are wide variations in the therapist's definition of the family constellation and the treatment unit. Some define families as including two genders who form a coalition as parents (Lidz). Many therapists include extended family members, since families are composed of two or more generations and generational boundaries are problems. Other therapists include family friendship relationships, persons related genetically and/or emotionally. It has been suggested that small children be omitted from on-going treatment sessions since abstract dialogue is misinterpreted and/or frightening to their precausal cognitive level.

Many family therapists devote the assessment sessions to gathering structural information by constructing a family chronology, drawing upon Toman's Family Constellation Theory and using generational transmission concepts for hypothesis formulations. Family chronologies have gained popularity with the advent of Roots on TV, making this task more interesting to the family members.

HOME TREATMENT

Families develop consensus experiences, distinctive views of their environment and family therapists frequently go to the home environment to do therapy, reversing the traditional professional territorial control. Reasons for home treatment are:

1. Family interactions are more natural and normal.
2. People play their everyday roles on their home ground.
3. It is easier to gather reluctant family members.
4. The family's own space is used.

Psychiatric nurses find family treatment easily adaptable to their professional practice techniques, since visiting homes is a familiar practice. More than any other professional, the nurse's presence in the home is accepted by the family. Family centered nursing concepts and public health experiences in the nurse's basic preparation give her many opportunities to become familiar with "healthy" families as well as family responses to stress and disease.

Just as there are preventive, acute and chronic areas of care, there are distinctions between the types and levels of family therapy on primary, secondary and tertiary levels.

Intensive family therapy is usually long-term, involving the working through of unconscious transference distortions in the family relationships with intrapsychic changes as the members resolve distortions about one another.

Supportive family therapy is usually short-term, with an approach aimed at clarifying communication, changing interaction patterns and helping families cope with concrete stress situations.

Sculpting family therapy is preventative therapy drawing on psychodrama and role playing to help family members become more sensitive and aware of one another, fostering role flexibility and openness.

Baseline criteria of adequate family interactions are (Koos):

1. Family members' personalities allow giving of emotional support and affection to each other.
2. The family provides for the basic needs of its members.
3. Each member accepts his roles and roles of others in the family (role interchangeability).
4. The family has a goal and is working toward that goal.
5. Family members are willing to accept the goals of the family as theirs and give up their individual goals for the family's goals.

The four major factors in family effectiveness are its productivity, leadership patterns, modes of expressing conflicts and the clarity of communication.

An economical classification of the diverse family therapy methods is by experiential and structured categories (Bowen). The experiential approach emphasizes subjective experiences of therapy; open, spontaneous relationships; the therapist's use of feelings and intuition and direct expression of feelings to others. The structured approach is a therapeutic method with a built-in blueprint to guide the course of therapy; the therapist's decisions are based on theory and stay on course with methods and goals.

COALITIONS, TRIANGULARIZATIONS AND CO-THERAPISTS

The concept of triangles describes the way two people relate to each other and involve others in emotional issues between them. A two-person system is basically unstable and the theory of triangularization holds that two people will predictably involve a third to make a triangle. Although this behavior is automatic and unconscious, the triangularization theory of both experiential and structured family therapists differs from Freud's family triangle Oedipal theory. The Oedipal complex has to do with sexual impulses, triangularization with two-person power coalitions (Caplow).

Two variables are important in triangling: the differentiation of self and the level of tension. The more tension exists, the more triangling occurs: the less ego differentiation the family member has, the more likely he is to be drawn into a coalition.

If a system involves four people, it becomes a series of interlocking triangles. In multi-personal systems, emotional problems may be acted out by three people with the others relatively uninvolved. When the central triangle in a family is modified, other family triangles are automatically modified and other members may not need to be involved in the therapy sessions.

A system of family therapy designed to modify triangular emotional states focuses on the central triangle in the family. The goal is to foster individualization and intellectual control over automatic emotional coalitions.

The use of co-therapists, or several therapists in the family therapy sessions, helps the therapist become aware of his over-involvement and automatic, unwitting entrance in the triangularization process.

EXPERIENTIAL FAMILY THERAPY

Family homeostasis is a pivotal concept of experiential therapy, implying bonds which are restrictive, impoverished and stereotyped. Homeostasis is the relatively stable state of equilibrium between the different, yet interdependent, family group members. Homeostasis operates on three levels: verbal exchanges, roles, and the family members' overt and covert needs.

Psuedo-mutuality and psuedo-hostility are terms used to describe family interaction restrictions which, in either positive or negative ways, limit the family's range of response by repetitious, non-productive stereotyped responses. These responses are as dangerous as the psuedo-mutual homeostasis which prohibits growth and differentiation.

Differentiation disturbances occur when boundaries are weak or tenuous between members. An undifferentiated family ego mass creates enmeshed families with gender and generation boundaries lacking. These family states are maintained by actions or transpersonal defenses, such as "mystification". Mystifications have three major dynamics:

1. Attribution - attributing a characteristic as "weak" or "bad" to implant a negative self-image.
2. Invalidation - the coercive invalidating or disqualifying of another's values, beliefs and thoughts.
3. Induction - the active recruitment of another person for collusive support.

Wynne and Singer have reported more than 40 actions, called communication deviances, that family members use in confusing, mystifying, and disorganizing one another.

The binding action to maintain homeostasis operates on the cognitive (ego) level, the dependency on the id level, and the loyalty and guilt on the superego level. Id-binding exploits the younger or weaker member's dependency and helplessness; ego-binding uses cognitive confusion and "double-bind" injunctions (Bateson); superego bindings are invisible loyalties that keep the member tied to the family or precipitate self-destructive acts for atonement.

In addition to binding, families use delegating and expelling as modes to maintain homeostasis and prevent the growth process of individualization and separation.

Intervention includes observing interactions and hurtful, nonsupportive exchanges. Tactics include unbinding, i.e., demystification, belated mourning, balancing of accounts and reconciliation across generations. The therapeutic process involves: developing trust with the family group; fostering awareness of the family's experiences; making new understandings of family transactions possible; helping the family in expressing and applying feelings; providing experiences for putting new actions and roles into use.

FAMILY COMMUNICATION

Satir identifies five basic roles family members assume to communicate their stress and pain. These "survival" stances, outcomes over time and "labels" are:

1. Placating (always agreeing)
   Outcome: digestive tract symptoms
   Label: simple neurosis
2. Blaming (belittling)
   Outcome: muscle, vessel constriction
   Label: aggressive, acting-out
3. Super reasonable (the computer)
   Outcome: drying up of the body's natural fluids
   Label: psychosomatic
4. Irrelevant (unrelated)
   Outcome: central nervous system pathology
   Label: psychosis
5. Congruent (leveling)
   Outcome: sharing, openness
   Label: none

Scapegoating, or labeling, is the embodiment of an evil force in a visible form. Once a behavior occurs, the person is labeled for rule breaking and soon accepts the role defined by the label. Parents thus give prescriptions or life scripts to their children. Scapegoating can be countered by developing a different value system for the person in the system - and in the system for the person.

STRUCTURED FAMILY THERAPY

Minuchin identifies a series of developmental tasks for the family related to the marriage, birth and development of children. Some of the tasks beginning at marriage are: the development of mutual accommodation, routines and patterns to regulate family life; shifting of loyalties from the family of origin and establishing extra familial relationships.

Tasks related to the birth of children include: task differentiation, developing subsystems and renegotiation of extended family boundaries.

Tasks related to the development of children focus on the adapting and restructuring of the family to accommodate the tasks and transitions of the unfolding personality.

Boundaries, the rules for defining who participates and for protecting differences within the system, are described on a continuum as clear, diffuse, rigid, affiliative, over affiliation and conflicting. Families provide their members identity, a sense of belonging and a sense of separateness. Generic and idiosyncratic transactional patterns regulate the family members' behavior. The therapist pinpoints transactional patterns and boundaries by constructing a "family map". The diagnosis is made by experience with, and observations of, the family's structure, flexibility, sensitivity, support and stress, developmental stage, and how symptoms are used to maintain the family's patterns. One of the most difficult tasks for the therapist is to avoid being drawn into supporting the system in its present state. To avoid this, it is suggested (Minuchin) that the therapist:

1. Obey family pathways but try to change the nature of the interaction.
2. Disobey the pathways and explicitly point to other interactions.
3. Disobey the pathways and explicitly request the use of other pathways.
4. Eliminate the pathways.

The therapist restructures the family by: marking boundaries, escalating stress, assigning tasks, utilizing symptoms, manipulating moods; supporting, educating and providing guidance. During reconstruction, the therapist acts as a catalyst to pinpoint conflicts and intervenes by showing the family other ways to relate to each other. Guidelines for the management of change (also applicable to other change experiences) which cause anger, discomfort and dispair (a "dislocation" phenomenon) include:

1. Anticipation of discomfort by anticipatory guidance, providing concrete examples.
2. Helping people anticipate the natural tendency to revert to former comfortable (yet nonproductive) interaction modes.
3. Shifting attention away from family members who are slower to change.

When family therapy is not contraindicated, either experiential or structured therapy can be effective. And for those individuals who do not wish family therapy, or who do not have families, there are many alternatives.

REVIEW QUESTIONS

1. What is homeostasis?
2. What strategies can the nurse use to avoid triangularization?
3. What are the contraindications for family therapy?
4. What are the seven stages of adult developmental and marital tasks?
5. What techniques and approaches do marriage therapists utilize?
6. How do structured and experiential family therapy theory and methods differ?

SUGGESTED REFERENCES

1. Bateson, G., et al.: A note on the double bind, Family Process II:154-161, 1963

2. Berman, E.M. and Lief, H.J.: Marital therapy from a psychiatric perspective: An overview, Am J Psychi VI:32-48, June, 1975

3. Bloch, D.A.: The clinical home visit, Seminars Psychi V:159-165, 1973

4. Boszormenyi-Nagi, J. and Spark, G.: Invisible Loyalties, Hagerstown, Md., 1973

5. Bowen, M.: Family therapy after 20 years, American Handbook of Psychiatry, Arieti, S., Ed., Treatment, Basic Books, New York, 2nd Ed., Vol. 5, pp. 367-392, 1975

6. Byasse, J.E. and Murrell, S.M.: Interaction patterns in families of autistic, disturbed and normal children, Am J Orthopsychi XLIII:473-483, April, 1975

7. Camp, H.: Structured family therapy: An outsider's perspective, Family Process, pp. 269-277

8. Carroll, E.: Family Therapy - Some observations and comparisons, Family Process III:178-185, March, 1964

9. Caplow, T.: Two Against One: Coalitions in Triad, Prentice Hall, Englewood Cliffs, N.J., 1969

10. Chase-Marshall, J.: Virginia Satir: Everybody's family therapist, Human Behavior XI:25-31, Sept., 1976

11. Chisholm, M.M., et al.: Psychiatric Community Mental Health Nursing Case Studies, Medical Examination Publishing Co., Inc., Flushing, N.Y., 1976

12. Faucett, J.: The family as a living open system: An emerging conceptual framework for nursing, International Nursing Review, Issue 202, pp. 113-118, July-Aug., 1974

13. Fitzgerald, R.F.: Conjoint Marital Therapy, Jason Aronson, New York, 1973

14. Fleck, S.: General systems approach to severe family psychology, Am J Psychi CXXXIII:669-673, June, 1976

15. Foley, V.: Introduction to Family Therapy, Grune & Stratton, New York, 1974

16. Francis, T.M.: Treatment in the home as a psychiatric nursing technique, In American Nurses Association, Clinical Sessions, Appleton-Century-Crofts, New York, pp. 286-295, 1968

17. GAP Report: Treatment of Families in Conflict: The Clinical Study of Family Process, The Committee on the Family Group for the Advancement of Psychiatry, Science House, New York, 1970

18. Greene, B.L.: A Clinical Approach to Marital Problems: Evaluation and Management, Charles C. Thomas, Publishers, Springfield, 1970

19. Guttman, H.A.: A contra indication for family therapy, Arch Gen Psychi XXIX:352-355, 1973

20. Hills, R. and Hansen, J.: Identification of conceptual frameworks utilized in family study, Marriage and Family Living XXII:279-311, 1960

21. Jacob, T.: Family interaction in disturbed and normal families: A methodological and substantive review, Psychological Bull LXXXIII:33-65, 1975

22. Koos, E.L.: The Sociology of the Patient, McGraw-Hill Book Co., New York, p. 67, 1959

23. Laing, R.D.: Mystification, confusion and conflict, In Boszarmenyi-Nagy, I. and Framo, J.L., Eds., Intensive Family Therapy, Harper & Row, New York, pp. 343-364, 1965

24. Lederer, W. and Jackson, D.D.: The Mirages of Marriage, W.W. Norton Co., New York, 1968

25. Levinson, D.J., et al.: The psychosocial development of men in early adulthood and the mid-life transition, In Ricks, D.F., Thomas, A. and Rott, M., Eds., Life History Research in Psychopathology, University of Minnesota Press, Minneapolis, Vol. 3, pp. 243-258, 1974

26. Lidz, T. and Fleck S.: The family: The developmental setting, In Arieti, S., Ed., American Handbook of Psychiatry, Basic Books, New York, Vol. I, pp. 252-263, 1974

27. McVicar, M.G. and Archibold, P.: A framework for family assessment in chronic illness, Nursing Forum XV:180-194, 1976

28. Minuchin, S.: Family and Family Therapy, Harvard University Press, Cambridge, 1974

29. Minuchin, S.: The use of an ecological framework in the treatment of a child, The Child and His Family, Anthony, E.J. and Koupernick, C., Eds., John Wiley & Sons, New York, pp. 41-57, 1970

30. Otto, H.: Has monogamy failed? Saturday Review, pp. 23-25, April 25, 1970

31. Samovilides, L.: Marital relationships: Frustration and fulfillment, Am J Psychoanal XXXIII:365-375, 1975

32. Satir, V., et al.: Helping Families to Change, Jason Aronson Co., New York, 1975

33. Searles, H.F.: The effort to drive the other person crazy - An element in the etiology and psychotherapy of schizophrenia, Br J Med Psychol XXXII:1-18, Jan., 1959

34. Skolnik, A.: Families can be unhealthy for children and other living things, Psychol Today V:18-22, 104-106, 1971

35. Smoyak, S., Ed.: The Psychiatric Nurse as Family Therapist, John Wiley-Biomedical Health Productions, New York, 1975

36. Speck, R. and Attneave, C.: Family Networks, Pantheon Press, New York, 1973

37. Starlin, H.: Separating Parents and Adolescents, Quadrangle Books, New York, 1974

38. Sussman, M.B.: The family systems in 1970's: Analysis, policies and programs, Family Health Care, Hymovich, D.P. and Barnard, M.U., Eds., McGraw-Hill Book Co., New York, pp. 18-37, 1973

39. Toman, W.: Family Constellation, Springer Publishing Co., New York, 1969

40. Waters, D.B.: Family therapy as a defense, J Am Acad Child Psychi XV:464-474, 1976

41. Wells, C.F. and Rabiner, E.: The conjoint family diagnostic interview and the family index of tension, Family Process, pp. 127-144, June, 1973

42. Weis, D.P.: Children's interpretation of marital conflict, Family Process XIII:385-393, Sept., 1974

43. Whitaker, C.: Psychotherapy of the absurd: With a special emphasis on the psychotherapy of aggression, Family Process XIV:1-16, March, 1975

44. Wynne, L.: Some indications and contraindications for exploratory family therapy, In Boszormenyi-Nagy, I. and Frano, J., Eds., <u>Intensive Family Therapy</u>, Harper & Row, New York, 1965

45. Wynne, L. and Singer, M.T.: Thought disorders and family relations of schizophrenias, I, A research strategy, <u>Arch Gen Psychi</u> IX:191-198, March, 1963; II, A classification of forms of thinking, <u>Arch Gen Psychi</u> IX:199-206, 1963

CHAPTER 18

ALTERNATIVE THERAPIES

Psychotherapy begins when a therapist is visited by a client with a problem who is seeking help to solve the problem. The client specifies the problem, verbally or nonverbally. The therapist must then respond and the response varies with the situation and the therapist's clinical orientation.

The problem situation has several facets: the problem itself, the client's insight into the problem, his affect and behavior and his ability to change. Different "schools of thought" may emphasize different facets. Psychoanalytic theorists emphasize insight while the behaviorists focus on behavior. Therapists who rely heavily upon drugs emphasize alteration of affect.

For the last 15 years a new group of therapists has offered "third force" alternatives with supportive therapies and with the human potential movement in which the therapeutic relationship is a direct and individual to individual one. The "third force" therapists emphasize the client's strengths and his ability to change. Secondly, they focus upon behavior, affect and insight.

Therapies may be one-to-one or in groups. Some therapists, as well as clients, prefer groups in which they do not fear emotional involvement with any single individual.

Unlike families, groups have no history, the members meet, form a group, members may leave, others join and eventually the group disbands. The "group" is peculiar to a specific time and a specific place. It cannot exist twice. Once terminated, the group may reform with the same members but it will not be the same.

In a given group, the members meet, exchange information, become involved, identify with the group and learn how their behaviors affect others. They express feelings, communicate openly and once the self-determination or autonomy of the group has been established, problems can be solved and individual changes can occur.

GROUP THERAPY

There are different types of groups:

1. Didactic groups. Group leader presents factual material for a guided discussion (adolescent sex education groups).
2. Therapeutic social clubs. Have parliamentary rules, elect officers, collect dues, plan activities. Increase skill in social participation. Especially good for outpatients.
3. Repressive-Inspirational groups. Build morale through strong identification and positive group emotions with inspirational talks, songs, recitals (AA and Synanon).

4. **Psychodrama.** Therapeutic controlled acting-out with three components:
   a. Common interactional matrix
   b. Common unconscious experiences
   c. Role reversal
   Excellent for children, adolescents, marriage and family problems.
5. **Free-Interaction groups.** Interactions lead to display of free and honest feelings, then to discussion, interpretation and changed behavior (Encounter or Sensitivity).

Some of the principles of group therapy are:

1. **Support.** Only group in society in which status is not based on personal attraction or achievement, but on an acknowledged need for help. Serves to protect the individual member.
2. **Stimulation.** Group stimulates verbalization and change by emotional contagion, affords opportunity to test out own problem with problems of others.
3. **Verbalization.** Group activities almost force expression of feelings. Shame will sometimes hamper an individual, group pressure will stimulate him.
4. **Practice.** Opportunity to practice new behaviors and test out old ones. Group will point out any problems.

Groups may be comprised of similar or dissimilar individuals. They are usually most productive when the members are similar enough to give support, yet different enough to expose each other to the stimulation of a variety of problems and ways of dealing with them.

Once the group members have been selected, the therapist enters into a working agreement with the patient which tells him:

1. What he can expect to gain from the group.
2. What is expected from him in the group.
3. What he can and cannot expect from the therapist.

Patients assume different roles within groups; some are positive and help build the group, others are negative. One of the therapist's major functions is to encourage constructive behaviors and to modify destructive ones.

Like people, groups have developmental stages:

1. **Formulative phase.** Deciding its primary goal and how to attain it. Communication stereotyped and restricted to socially acceptable interchanges.
2. **Working phase.** Recognizable when communication turns to negative confrontation. Establish a group hierarchy and group cohesiveness emerges. Work until goals are met or group is terminated.
3. **Termination phase.** Not a happy time; members will need support to close in an orderly positive way.

Groups may use psychoanalytic techniques or transactional analysis or other ways to analyze or interpret the group dynamics and process.

Groups may range from nude marathon groups to sensitivity training groups to life change groups.

Just as some therapists prefer group therapy to individual therapy, other therapists prefer crisis intervention to more extended therapy.

CRISIS INTERVENTION

Crises can't wait to be analyzed. They need immediate resolution. The client asks for, and wants, decisions and solutions. Although described in terms of external events: death, marriage, loss of job, illness, etc., crises exist only within the perception of the individual who must adapt to a significant change in role or in self-concept within a certain time limit. After the first impact, the individual experiences increasing tension with disorganized or uncharacteristic behavior. He may be able to adapt and resolve the problem or he may become increasingly disorganized and fail to solve the problem.

Crisis intervention helps such individuals (or families) to prevent maladaptive behavior and prevent frank psychotic breaks. Clinically, crisis intervention is time limited (usually 5-10 sessions), immediate (as close to crisis event as possible) and actively focused on the current problem. Instead of interpreting, the therapist responds to manifest content. However, to make the decisions necessary, the therapist needs to have clinical experience, to understand causes and to have a feel for how the past influences the present behavior.

For the flexible, experienced, sophisticated nurse who thrives on emergency situations, the crisis center is a challenge.

Crises can't wait to be analyzed, but need to be resolved fast. The patient usually asks and wants decisions and solutions. It is an error to be directive in a crisis for several reasons:

1. The solution may not be best for the patient.
2. The patient may not like the consequences of the solution.
3. A masochist will make sure the decision turns out wrong.
4. Decisions from others always foster dependency.

The only way to assist a patient in crisis is to:

1. Help him consider his alternatives.
2. Help him assess the consequences of his alternatives.

Any individual is faced with many decisions in his life. He makes these decisions by using habitual mechanisms and coping reactions. In a crisis situation, he is faced with a problem that he can't resolve with his habitual techniques, or within the expected time limit.

If he can try new measures and meet the crisis, he emerges with greater strength and an enhanced self-image. If he cannot meet the crisis by making a decision, he will feel greater anxiety and stress. Latent conflicts are stimulated, new symptoms are generated, and he seeks help.

Because he seeks help he is more amenable to alter old patterns or develop new ones of a more adaptive nature. Crises are of two kinds:

1. Developmental - marriage, death, etc., common to all.
2. Situational - illness, accidents, loss of job, or other random events.

Crises have limits in time. They can't last too long for no one can survive without disintegrating. Crisis intervention, therefore, must be brief and it must be immediate to intervene in the process of mental decompensation.

Crisis theory assumes that the individual in crisis can be "turned around", and that neither he nor the therapist has time for insights into causes, that handling the patient's reaction to the crisis is more important than understanding the dynamics of the crisis. Crisis theory is reality-oriented and its basic purposes are to:

1. Avoid hospitalization.
2. Maintain patient's functioning within his family and community.
3. Assist in problem solving.
4. Facilitate emotional growth.

The nurse may meet the patient in a crisis at a clinic, mental health center, home, emergency room, or elsewhere. He may be there voluntarily or because someone brought him. The steps in crisis intervention are similar to the steps in noncrisis situations, but are, of necessity, truncated:

1. Initial contact - the nurse must convince the patient that help is available.
2. Presenting symptoms - the patient will focus on whatever is bothering him, and treatment starts where he is at the moment.
3. Background - the nurse should obtain as much factual data as possible about the family, the patient's medical status, and then the crisis:
   a. Crisis as identified by patient.
   b. Cause as he identifies it.
   c. His attempts to solve it.
   d. His expectations for help in solving it.
4. Interventions - the nurse has the advantage because the individual:
   a. Can't stand the stress much longer,
   b. Needs her help,
   c. Wants her help,
   and she will seek to intervene by helping him look at options, choose one, and act on it.

A crisis situation can be a "turning point" experience in anyone's life and it can increase his ability to control or adapt to his environment.

As in most cases of extreme emotional distress, the identification of the focal problem may require an exploratory dialogue. The real problem may or may not be what the patient has focused on but prompt attention to the problem the patient identifies will alleviate his immediate stress.

Crisis intervention therapy is immediate. Although the crisis center nurse needs experience to draw on, self-confidence to sustain her, and enough flexibility to see many options - it is usually the new nurse who finds herself working in this area because older nurses don't want it. She can learn as much as the patient from the crisis situation, and may welcome the opportunity to work in crisis intervention.

The psychiatric team in the crisis or community center may no longer have well-defined roles. The relationship is more collegial and the members do what they do best or whatever needs to be done at the moment. Except for purely legal functions, the roles no longer exist as they did. The members work together and trust each other. The nurse may do therapy, the psychologist may be the administrator, and the psychiatrist is no longer in the role of the omnipotent leader.

The crisis center may confine itself to specific problems: suicide prevention center, drug addiction center, rape center.

The nurse who is not comfortable with the typical group therapies or in crisis intervention, may prefer one of the more recent alternatives, referred to as the human potential therapies.

HUMAN POTENTIAL

The human potential proponents also like brief present-oriented encounters. They focus upon change and, as Rouslin says: "There is also the inherent idea that a person is forever a tabula rasa with either no prior internalized experience, or no experience that can't be eradicated by performance of the prescribed ritual".

REALITY THERAPY

All disturbed people have two things in common:

1. They can't meet all of their basic needs.
2. They refuse to face reality.

Some degree of denial is utilized by all patients. To lead them back to reality a therapist needs to:

1. Help them face the real world.
2. Help them meet their needs in the real world.

People have the same needs but do not have the same ability to satisfy them. In order to satisfy needs, two things must be present:

1. The individual has to be involved with at least one other person.
2. The other person has to be able to face reality and satisfy his own needs.

Until a patient can form an active relationship with someone in a more effective way than he now does, he won't be able to satisfy his needs.

The need for identity is the most important of all needs and must be fulfilled. The two paths to identify need fulfillment are:

1. The need to give and receive love.
2. The need to feel worthwhile to self and to others.

They do not necessarily go together. Being loved may not make anyone feel worthwhile. To feel worthwhile requires satisfactory behavior patterns. If the needs are not met, they will remain a problem.

When anyone comes for psychiatric help, he can't meet his needs because he lacks a person who cares about him and whom he cares about. Fulfilling those needs has nothing to do with the past; he has to do it in the present.

Needs have to be satisfied in ways that do not prevent others from meeting their own needs. Patients are people who have lost - or never had - the ability to meet their needs. They are called irresponsible instead of ill.

Therapy is a form of teaching involving three separate procedures:

1. Involvement - therapist must become involved with patient so he can begin to face reality.
2. Rejection - therapist must reject patient's unrealistic behavior but maintain the involvement.
3. Teaching - therapist teaches better ways to meet needs within reality.

Involvement is the most difficult step, but until there is involvement, there is no therapy.

Differences Between Reality Therapy and Conventional Therapy:

Conventional	Reality
1. Mental illness exists and can be classified.	1. Mental illness doesn't exist and everyone is responsible for his own behavior.
2. Patient can change once he understands his past problem.	2. Present is important. Past can't be changed nor does it limit anyone.

3. Transference must occur.

3. Relate to patients as "self" not as transference figure.

4. Must gain insight into unconscious mind in order to change.

4. Patient can't excuse behavior because of unconscious motivations.

5. Will not say behavior is good or bad.

5. Emphasize morality of behavior, face issue of right and wrong.

6. Don't teach people to behave better, they will learn when they understand their unconscious conflicts.

6. Teach better ways to fulfill needs.

Reality therapy requires a strong yet sensitive therapist who can become emotionally involved with every patient. It is effective with patients who are "irresponsible".

TRANSACTIONAL ANALYSIS (TA)

Reality therapy recognizes identity as the basic need. TA identifies three needs: the need for strokes (recognition or physical contact), the need to structure time (for oneself or for others - called leadership), and the need for excitement.

Most of one's time is spent structuring time as excitingly as possible or in seeking the leadership of others to help in structuring it. Some of the more exciting ways to structure time is with past-times, rituals and games. Rituals are formally prescribed ways of getting through social situations in accordance with the rules of "one's own kind". All the right people have the same rituals, outsiders do not. Once the "in-group" has been joined, certain people are selected with whom one wishes to spend more time. Those selected have the same past-times (hobbies, life styles, interests). Unfortunately, rituals and past-times are designed to control situations, not to arouse emotions or to excite.

Games provide excitement. Games are actually a series of "duplex" transactions (on two different levels of communication at once) and they have an unexpected payoff such as guilt, rage or depression. These payoff feelings are called stamps. The kind of stamps collected defines one's racket, i.e., the depression racket, the guilt racket, etc.

An individual's games and racket are closely associated with his life script. The script is a decision made by the person himself, but made at a very early age with an inadequate or biased data base. The data are based on early interactions with others from which one learns the basic four life positions:

I'm OK	You're OK
I'm OK	You're not OK
I'm not OK	You're OK
I'm not OK	You're not OK

On the basis of one of these positions, the life script decision as to how he will spend his life is made.

These positions are learned before the ego states have matured. There are three ego states: Parent, Child and Adult. All three ego stages are present in adults, but the Child and the Parent dictate adherence to the life script, while the Adult can decide to stop playing games and seek help to change his racket.

The Child represents the early feelings and behaviors, joys and freedom of childhood, the Parent represents the advice, values prohibitions of the parents, the Adult is the computer that gathers data, programs expectancies and makes decisions. Games involve communication from Child to Parent and Parent to Child instead of from Adult to Adult in an adult transaction. There are other combinations also.

Once the individual seeks assistance through TA he is bound by a contractual agreement. He specifies exactly what he wants to achieve in the relationship, the therapist accepts or refuses the contract depending upon his opinion as to his ability to assist in achieving the contractual objectives.

TA is useful to the individual as a "do-it-yourself" therapy but is most effective in the group situation. It is effective with the mentally retarded as well as with alcoholics and juvenile delinquents.

RATIONAL EMOTIVE THERAPY (RET)

Alcoholics and sexually inadequate individuals respond well to Rational Emotive Therapy. RET is most effective with groups whose members all have the same problems. RET is a cognitively oriented therapy although it stresses the affective and motor aspects as well.

RET emphasizes the fact that man is a rational being. What happens to an individual is not important but the individual's reaction to the event is important. His reaction is cognitive and emotional and based upon an irrational Belief System. When the Activating event (A) is followed by a highly charged emotional Consequence (C), C is not caused by A but by B (the Belief System). When these irrational Beliefs can be Disputed (D) by rational challenges, the disturbed C eventually ceases to exist.

RET holds that virtually all serious emotional problems stem from an irrational belief system. It is important for an individual to understand that his dysfunctional emotional Consequences (C) are not caused by the prior Activating event (A) of his life but by his unrealistic Beliefs (B). He is the cause of his own problems. Once the individual discovers Insight No. 1: that his self-defeating be-

havior is related to his faulty Belief system and not to past and
present Activating events; and Insight No. 2: that, while he may
have made himself disturbed in the past, he is disturbed now because he is reinforcing his Beliefs and reindoctrinating himself; he
is ready to develop Insight No. 3: that Insight No. 1 and Insight No.
2 are not enough and he needs help.

The Rational Emotive Therapy that he seeks will be highly cognitive,
active, directive, discipline-oriented and includes homework assignments. RET is a method of quickly changing personality by facing
irrational beliefs, "should" systems and by actively enhancing the
more human side of one's nature.

GESTALT THERAPY

Unlike the other therapies, Gestalt deals only with the Now. Present-oriented, the need-fulfillment pattern is here seen as a process
of Gestalt formation and destruction. To the external perceptions
are added the Gestalten that form in the body and in the individual's
relationship to his environment.

Needs activate behavior both perceptually and motorically and activities to satisfy the needs are carried out. This process, constantly
being repeated, is described as the progressive formation and destruction of perceptual and motor gestalts. When the process is going well, figure and ground are sharply differentiated. The
individual's figures (needs) dominate the field and his motor and
perceptual behaviors are concentrated on one particular thing. The
experiencing of needs and failures to fulfill them is apparent in
therapy in nonverbal behavior, lack of interest, confusion and repetitive behavior.

The process fails because there is: (1) poor perceptual contact with
the environment or with the body itself; (2) blocking of open expression of needs; and (3) repression of Gestalten formation. The therapist tries to break up a poorly organized field and to accentuate each
emerging figure. If the figure is blocked the therapist tries to unblock the impulse so it can reorganize the field. He does this by
focusing on "What are you doing that interferes with your meeting
your needs at this moment"? He needs to be sensitive to body language and to help the client become aware of it also. Therapy can
only be done in the "NOW". Therapy deals, not with the inner
depths, but with the outermost surfaces, to observe, to "see" what
is going on. Neurotics find it difficult to see in this way, to be in
touch with themselves.

Gestalt therapy identifies five layers of neurosis:

1. Phony layer - (top-dog/under-dog and other game playing to
   avoid facing unpleasant experiences).
2. Phobic layer - (resistance to being what we are, to discovering
   life).
3. Impasse - unable to use own resources and environmental support is unavailable).

4. Implosive layer - (feeling of nothing, of being a mere thing, of being dead).
5. Explosive layer - (expression of four types of explosion: joy, grief, orgasm and anger).

To be authentic, one must progress through all layers and have all four avenues of explosion available. Gestalt therapy is most useful in groups and in crisis intervention. Full resolution of crises (or other impasses) requires being processed or having conditioned behavior patterns made conscious and then changed, being able to say good-bye (finish the situation), being able to give up the resentments associated with the behavior patterns and allowing oneself to experience. Recognizing one's feelings is not enough, experiencing them is a necessary step.

Many more alternatives to analysis and behavior modification have been developed in the last 10 years: Arica (physical and mental exercises to unblock conditioning and allow experiencing of self), Guided Fantasy (developing strengths and insights by visualizing imaginary structured scenes), EST (Erhardt Seminar Training focuses on a meaningless world and 60 hours of training in how to experience yourself and improve your own world).

Esthetic therapies are also available but are not therapies in the same sense the preceding ones are. Poetry therapy, dance therapy, music therapy and art therapy can all be effective whether or not patients are artistic or have rhythm.

REVIEW QUESTIONS

1. What is reality therapy?
2. What is a transaction?
3. Which alternative therapies are used with alcoholics?
4. How do reality therapy and rational-emotive therapy differ?
5. How do the "third force" therapies differ from the analytic therapies?
6. What is a gestalt?
7. What are some of the principles of group therapy?
8. What are the developmental stages of groups?
9. What is the underlying theory of crisis intervention?
10. What are the principles of crisis theory?
11. How is crisis intervention accomplished?

SUGGESTED REFERENCES

1. Barlotucci, G. and Drayer, C.: An overview of crisis intervention in the emergency room, Am J Psychi CXXX:953-960, Sept., 1973

2. Berne, E.: Games nurses play, Am J Nursing CXXII:483-487, March, 1972

3. Berne, E.: Games People Play, Grove Press, Inc., New York, 1964

4. Berne, E.: Principles of Group Treatment, Oxford University Press, New York, 1966

5. Berne, E.: The Structure and Dynamics of Organizations and Groups, Grove Press, Inc., New York, 1963

6. Berne, E.: Transactional Analysis in Psychotherapy, Grove Press, Inc., New York, 1961

7. Bry, A., Ed.: Inside Psychotherapy, Basic Books, Inc., New York, 1972

8. Bry, A.: The TA Primer, Harper & Row, New York, 1973

9. Fagan, J. and Shepherd, I.L., Eds.: Gestalt Therapy Now, Harper Colophon Books, New York, 1970

10. Feder, S.: Maturational factors in self-referral to experiential groups, J Am Psychoanalytic Assoc XXI:851-866, 1973

11. Getty, C. and Shay, C.: Co-therapy as an egalitarian relationship, Am J Nursing LXIX:767-771, April, 1969

12. Glasser, W.: Reality Therapy, Harper & Row, Publishers, New York, 1965

13. Goldberg, C.: Group sensitivity training, International J Psychi, Aronson, J., Ed., Science House, New York, Vol. IX, pp. 165-232, 1970

14. Harris, T.A.: I'm OK-You're OK, Harper & Row, Publishers, New York, 1967

15. James, M.and Jongeward, D.: Born to win, Transactional Analysis with Gestalt Experiments, Addison-Wesley Publishing Co., Reading, Mass., 1971

16. Levic, M.: Art in psychotherapy, In Current Psychiatric Therapies, Masserman, J., Ed., Grune & Stratton, New York, pp. 93-99, 1975

17. Lewin, K.K.: Brief Psychotherapy, Warren H. Green, Inc., St. Louis, 1970

18. Marram, G.D.: The Group Approach in Nursing Practice, C.V. Mosby Co., St. Louis, 1973

19. Meitzell, J. and Kornreich, M.: It works, Psychol Today V: 57-61, 1971

20. Meyer, V. and Chesser, E.J.: Behavior Therapy in Clinical Psychiatry, Science House, New York, 1970

21. Perls, F.S.: Gestalt Therapy Verbatim, Real People Press, Lafayette, Calif., 1969

22. Perls, F.S.: In and Out of the Garbage Pail, Real People Press, Lafayette, Calif., 1969

23. Pietropinto, A.: Poetry therapy in groups, Current Psychiatric Therapies, Masserman, J., Ed., pp. 221-232, 1975

24. Rogers, C.R.: Encounter Groups, Harper & Row, New York, 1970

25. Romano, M.D.: Sexual counseling in groups, J Sex Research IX:69-78, Feb., 1973

26. Rouslin, S.: Commentary on the new "therapies", Perspectives Psychi Care XII:59, 1976

27. Rouslin, S.: Relatedness in group psychotherapy, Perspectives Psychi Care XI:165-171, 1973

28. Schloss, G.: Psychopoetry, Grosset & Dunlap, New York, 1976

29. Whitaker, D.S. and Lieberman, M.A.: Psychotherapy Through the Group Process, Atherton Press, New York, 1970

30. Yalom, I.D.: The Theory and Practice of Group Psychotherapy, Basic Books, Inc., New York, 1970

CHAPTER 19

INSTITUTIONAL THERAPIES

Hospitalization for "mental illness" has been a practice for many years, and before hospitalization, the "queer", "violent", "bedeviled", cr "sick" individual was often isolated in some way from family and community.

The Community Mental Health Act of 1964 provides for the construction of community mental health centers and mandates that such a community mental health center must serve a given "community" of people, be accessible to them, and provide 10 state services. The last five services:

6. Diagnostic services.
7. Rehabilitation.
8. Pre-care and after-care.
9. Training programs for professionals and nonprofessionals.
10. Research and evaluation.

are designed to support and implement the first five services which each individual community mental health center must provide:

1. Inpatient treatment.
2. Outpatient treatment.
3. Partial hospitalization.
4. Emergency services 24 hours per day.
5. Consultation and education services available to community agencies and professional individuals.

These five services must be fully functional before the other services are added.

Since 1955, the emphasis in patient treatment has been shifting from inpatient to outpatient facilities. The average daily hospital census is down, the duration of stay is shorter and the number of outpatients has increased. However, hospital admissions have increased, largely due to the high rate of readmissions.

INPATIENT FACILITIES

Inpatient care has traditionally been available in three areas: public mental hospitals, general hospitals, and private psychiatric hospitals.

When the equilibrium between the needs of the individual and the needs of the environment cannot be maintained, it becomes necessary to intervene in the situation and remove the individual to a different environment.

Some individuals who cannot function in one community function quite well in another and hospitalization is not required.

The actively self-destructive individual is often hospitalized to protect him. The actively aggressive and dangerous individual is often hospitalized to protect the community.

Hospitalization can be an emergency measure when outpatient facilities fail. Hospitalization can also be the only way that chronic psychotic patients are able to receive therapeutic help. Hospitalization also provides for complicated medical treatments, somatic therapy, or milieu therapy that cannot be carried out for an individual in any other way. The functions of hospitalization are thus three:

1. Protective-custodial
   a. Protection of patient
   b. Protection of community
   c. Change of environment
2. Diagnostic
   a. Special medical procedures
   b. Closer continuous observation
3. Therapeutic
   a. Remotivation of patient and family to change life styles and behavior
   b. Pharmacotherapy with complicated routines, or potentially toxic drugs, and to be certain drugs are taken
   c. Somatic therapy such as ECT
   d. Social-personal-familial therapy to help patient develop social and peer relationships, or to look at his own behavior, without family interference

The psychiatric unit of a general hospital may carry less stigma for an individual patient and he may be willing to be admitted to the unit when he would refuse to enter a private or public psychiatric hospital.

Some of the existing psychiatric units are physically a part of the hospital but separate in every other way. A psychiatric team involved on such a unit loses much of its usefulness by such separation and the general hospital loses more. No general hospital is capable of providing the best medical care unless psychiatric services are available. One of the primary functions of the psychiatric team then is to provide consultant services for all patients.

This psychiatric unit should have all the treatment methods available in a psychiatric hospital: psychotherapy, somatic therapy, social services, occupational therapy, recreational therapy.

The private psychiatric hospital is usually able to provide a larger staff and more individualized therapy. It can usually display comforts, luxuries, and facilities unobtainable in any other care center.

Many private hospitals focus upon a particular type of patient or program and have many advantages as centers for treating alcoholics, drug addicts, children or adolescents.

The private and public hospitals may emphasize different environmental and therapeutic factors but they should both have:

1. Medical care facilities.
2. Laboratory facilities to follow-up drug effects and avoid complications.
3. Physical facilities for individual or group therapy.
4. Professional psychiatric teams with members representing psychiatry, psychology, nursing, and social work.
5. Professional personnel and facilities for occupational therapy (OT) and recreational therapy (RT).
6. Libraries.
7. Some provision for religious support for patients who wish it and can tolerate it.

The public mental hospital is often maligned, ridiculed, and scorned. Even the nomenclature is disparaging for the literature refers to private psychiatric hospitals but public mental hospitals.

However these hospitals have functioned in the past, they are now being modernized and more adequately staffed. For the patient who cannot afford the economic stress of private or general hospital rates; for the patient who needs a structured environment that doesn't insist that he get well in a hurry; or for the patient whose condition is too advanced or irreversible, the public hospital may be the facility of choice.

Some of the problems inherent in public institutional care can be traced to geographic locations. Public hospitals have often been located in communities or inner city areas from which competent psychiatric teams could not be recruited. When the team members came from a distance, were separated from family and friends, and sometimes from many social activities, they formed inbred groups with rigid structures. Instead of being a bridge between the patient and the outside world, the "group" became a gap that increased the patient's feelings of alienation and served to intensify or increase the pathological processes.

Other problems may be related to the hospital subcultures involving the patient in a completely unrealistic milieu. The "cult of psyche", or the "catharsis cult", or the cult of "accepting me as I am" focus on the patient's symptoms, feelings, desires. Behavior is discussed, interpreted, reinterpreted and then discussed, again. A "deviant" milieu in which patients may spend months in discussions of their sexual practices, their respective family members or mates, instead of a milieu emphasizing social intercourse and personal strengths, leads to a pattern that makes adjustment to an outside world that de-emphasizes these behaviors most difficult.

Hospital subcultures can also teach patients which behaviors are rewarded or punished by discharge or readmission. Some patients develop a life style of commitment whenever a change or "vactation" from problems is desired.

One of the advantages of a public hospital is the opportunity to establish a therapeutic community with a large group of patients. A therapeutic community is "milieu therapy" and the entire stay is treatment time and everything that happens to a patient is part of the treatment program.

Every detail of hospital life is integrated into a continuous program of treatment. Part of the program must necessarily be the appeal of the physical grounds, of the interior decor, of the food. The behavior of all the personnel becomes part of the program.

All activities are organized with regard to their greatest therapeutic effectiveness. Social interventions are planned and there is no emphasis on a pleasant stay; if the situations are sometimes stressful, the patient will not suffer and may, in fact, respond positively.

Changes can be accomplished not only by means of formal therapy but also by means of corrective emotional experiences in various activity programs. Recreational Therapy (RT) is important for play fulfills important psychological needs such as exuberance, joy in activity, rules and structure that are not permanent or punitive. Occupational Therapy (OT) serves as a transitional step between recreation and "serious" work. The type of task a patient selects, the way he accomplishes it, and his mode of self-expression may be of diagnostic or prognostic value.

Direction to the therapeutic program is usually given by a psychiatrist. He works with all members of the team and integrates their skills and activities. The emotional climate among members of the team affects the outcomes of hospital treatment. A positive, cohesive, functioning team in which the members support and implement each other can provide positive experiential learning.

Strife within the psychiatric team is upsetting to patients and they may behave negatively or manipulate the members by playing one against the other. Frequent staff meetings help maintain the therapeutic milieu by giving team members some understanding of the skills of others and show them how they implement each other.

Daily rounds are not practical in a public psychiatric institution. Group meetings on the ward are not only time-saving but afford opportunities lacking in rounds:

1. Administrative problems can be considered.
2. The patients have a chance to know each other.
3. The patients can learn to know the members of the team - and members as a team.
4. The team members have a chance to know the patients.
5. A sense of community develops.

Ward meetings serve the same function as other group therapies:

1. Help the patient free himself of immature attitudes and behaviors.
2. Help him strengthen his own inner controls.
3. Help him negotiate his inner conflicts.

The psychiatric team in the public institution does not have as much blurring of roles as occurs in the community or private structures. Traditionally:

1. The psychiatrist - directs care, provides therapy for the patient, may also work with the family in therapy, and integrates data from other members.
2. The psychologist - does the clinical testing and provides psychometric data for the team.
3. The social worker - works with the family and patient in the external setting, in areas of family assistance, foster home placement, vocational rehabilitation and brings family history data to the team.
4. The nurse - gives nursing care, especially in the somatic therapies, observes patients' behaviors in a close interpersonal situation and brings descriptive observational data to the team.

These roles are changing and are becoming less differentiated and more interchangeable.

Other professionals and nonprofessionals contribute in their own ways. Occupational and recreational therapists may provide the most significant data in staff meetings. The people who have the most contact with the patients - the psychiatric aides - are being better trained and helped to offer their own observational data to the team and to participate actively in the planning and execution of the patients' care.

On the whole, the nurse who works in a public institution can expect to find:

1. A fairly structured caste system with the administration on top and the patient on the bottom.
2. Severely ill psychotic patients rather than mildly neurotic ones.
3. A "chronic" orientation and some degree of pessimism on the part of staff.
4. Staff who are not accustomed to having nurses run things.
5. Varying degrees of rigidity and control on the part of most of the staff.

The nurse who wishes to bring some positive change to public hospital care needs first to listen and allow herself to be "sized-up" by the personnel. Once accepted into the subculture, she can begin to change the subculture by:

1. Rearranging furniture so that eye contact and communication are facilitated.

2. Paint and/or decorate the wards whenever possible. Patients and staff who work together in such efforts - both planning and executing - develop a new relationship and new self-concepts.
3. Patients can braid rugs in OT, make new furniture, or any number of other things.
4. Mirrors and calendars when available and not contraindicated are most effective methods to reinforce reality.
5. Plants and fish are decorative, provide a new topic for conversation, and give patients nonthreatening things to care about and care for.

In addition to changing the physical environment, the nurse can establish staff groups for "inservice education" in how to change custodial care habits to individualized therapeutic care. She can do this by:

1. Giving factual information on development and behavior.
2. Demonstrating techniques of observation and communication.
3. Encouraging the staff to observe and record patient behaviors.
4. Stressing that "behavior has meaning" and "behavior can be changed".
5. Helping the staff re-educate patients in the basic behaviors of: incontinence, social graces including eating habits, and personal appearance.

Before trying to institute too much "remotivation", the nurse would be wise to assure herself that regression processes have been halted enough for the patient to participate.

Behavior therapy is useful in changing habit patterns especially for rewarding and reinforcing acceptable social behaviors.

The nurse who has worked on an inpatient unit may find it difficult to adjust to working in the community. If she is desirous of changing her job, it might be easier for her to shift to a partial hospitalization facility.

For the patient who requires closer observation than is possible on an outpatient basis, part-time hospitalization is appropriate. He can be removed from a stressful environment, participate in the therapeutic milieu, yet maintain contacts with his social group.

Partial hospitalization may enable a patient to continue working. It is much more economical for both patient and community. Partial hospitalization may refer to day, night, or weekend facilities.

The day hospital has been in existence since the late forties. It can serve different functions and may be:

1. A definitive treatment center.
2. A transitional facility between hospitalization and community - going in either direction.
3. An extended outpatient clinic.
4. A center for special programs such as vocational rehabilitation or somatic therapy, or for care of emotionally disturbed children.

Any given day hospital may serve more than one function and usually does. At a day hospital, the patient can be provided a full program of observation, treatment, and care.

Unlike the public hospital, the attitude in a day hospital is one of optimism - the patient is expected to get better quickly and the staff and the patient will work as partners in the process of getting better.

His behavior is viewed as being his own responsibility; he needs to recognize his own condition and come for treatment before he needs emergency care.

Legally defined, one day of partial hospitalization is equal to six hours of care. Therefore, day hospitals usually provide services Monday through Friday from 9:00 A.M. to 3:00 P.M. The patient can receive all the benefits of hospitalization, yet return to his family during the evenings, nights, and on weekends.

The evening and weekend hospitals use the same space and facilities as the day hospital. Two evenings a week is the usual procedure and two groups of patients can be accommodated on Monday/Wednesday or Tuesday/Thursday from 6:00 P.M. to 9:00 P.M. or on Saturdays from 9:00 A.M. to 3:00 P.M.

The evening hospital is well suited for patients who:

1. Have left the day hospital but need a little more support.
2. Have not yet had to interrupt their usual daytime activities.

The weekend hospital may be the best solution for patients who live at a distance, and it provides more intensive care than outpatient facilities, yet doesn't interfere with family life.

The weekend hospital may provide care on both Saturday and Sunday or only on Saturday, depending upon the facility. It is usually only one day.

The night hospital allows patients to work during the day and receive treatment and participate in the therapeutic milieu during the night - usually from 12:00 midnight to 6:00 A.M. Monday through Friday. The night hospital helps people who:

1. Are able to work but can't adapt to a traumatic home situation.
2. Are able to work but have trouble with self-control during leisure time, such as alcoholics.

Evening and night hospitals are not as numerous as day hospitals. The programs offered may differ in different communities but in order to benefit from any of the programs, the client needs to have a meaningful activity during the day. An evening or night hospital is useful near college campuses and is effective with students who are occupied with school during the day but need help or support at other times.

The nurse used to the long-term or comparatively lengthy hospital stay in a public institution is faced with a mobile population who come and go as they wish. She will need to compress 24 hours of activity into six. In order to achieve the desired behavioral outcomes for her nursing therapy she must:

1. Identify goals faster.
2. Choose the alternative most effective for a given patient at a given time.

In essence, the nurse involved with partial hospitalization needs to have had some experience to draw on, to use in planning and implementing her plan of therapy.

The patient is subject to a variety of stresses not encountered by the hospitalized patient. He goes in and out of the community and needs support and encouragement to face the problems and keep moving out. The nurse will have to be:

1. Flexible (to react with changing situations).
2. Perceptive (to read the ward atmosphere).
3. Realistic (to recognize, and be ready to modify, the effect that patients who are coming in and going out have on the ones who are staying).

Once she is competent in dealing with partial hospitalization, the nurse can move into the outpatient facilities.

OUTPATIENT FACILITIES

Since one of the major goals of psychiatric treatment is to increase the patient's ability to run his own life, outpatient care is preferred whenever possible.

A patient, no matter how much subjective tension he feels, can be considered for outpatient care if he:

1. Functions socially with reasonable effectiveness.
2. Sleeps at least five to six hours a night.
3. Has no problems with eating habits that would lead to weight loss.
4. Understands instructions and is willing and able to follow them.

Some of these criteria can be ignored if a patient's family can supervise him during critical times.

Even severe delusional or perceptual disturbances or preoccupation with suicidal thoughts do not rule out the patient as a candidate for the outpatient services. If outpatient facilities prove insufficient to maintain the patient, he may try partial or full hospitalization.

Outpatient clinics focus on prevention in all its aspects:

1. Primary prevention - reducing or eradicating mental health disorders (crisis intervention).

2. Secondary prevention - reducing or ameliorating the duration of disease or condition through early detection and treatment (ECT).
3. Tertiary prevention - reducing or limiting impairment or irreversible conditions which may result from the disease and to begin rehabilitation process (psychotherapy).

Outpatient care focuses on brief psychotherapies that have a predetermined beginning and end.

The patient is faced with certain expectations which are not set so high that he cannot meet them. His clinic and home visits and his therapy are individualized. He will probably visit with his therapist one hour a week - same time, same day, same place, if possible.

The greater the expectation that he will attain the goal, and the more important the goal, the more likely it is that the patient will try to attain it and to listen and act on relevant information from others on how to attain it.

In 1967, Yale instituted a "three-day hospitalization" plan with time-limited contracts and intensive intervention. The client was guaranteed three days of inpatient treatment and 30 days of outpatient follow-up. The time-limit facilitated rapid identification of problems and expectations that the patient would be ready for discharge in three days. The staff was more optimistic and both staff and family saw the patient as not hopeless and not there for just custodial care. At the one-year follow-up of the first 100 patients, 63 percent had not been rehospitalized (Feirstein).

More and more the nurse is becoming an active, essential team member; her function as a co-therapist is increasingly important.

The nurse's presence is usually reassuring to a patient, and his faith in her often makes the nurse the most significant person in his therapy. She is not often viewed with the hostility directed at psychiatrists, psychologists, and social workers. She still retains the traditional functions of physical care, observation, and nurturance. More than any other member of the team, she controls the milieu.

MILIEU THERAPY

Milieu therapy considers the patient's needs in relation to the needs of the group. The word itself refers to what is essentially a growth-promoting environment for patients. It rests on a sound understanding of psychodynamics. The atmosphere created is primarily accomplished by the nursing staff.

The therapeutic milieu can be accomplished by:

1. Environmental manipulation:
   a. Regulating the patient's physical space. The amount of geographic freedom allowed a patient is arrived at after an assessment of his individual needs, his drives, his defenses, his strengths, his energy, his physical condition, and his vulnerability.

   b. Regulating the patient's interpersonal contacts. They are
      regulated in accordance with the therapeutic objectives pro-
      posed by the team for the patient. To go back into society,
      he has to be able to resume old relationships at some level
      and has to learn to cope in this area.
2. Attitude therapy: Most effective when staff concentrates on one
   principal line of approach at a time. Attitudes involve three related components:
   a. Emotional responses. Vary with the personalities involved
      and the immediate circumstances. Any prescribed attitude
      involves only positive feelings (the negative feelings are
      brought under control), and how the feelings are shown to the
      patients. A patient with involutional melancholia might re-
      act well to warm friendliness, a paranoid patient would mis-
      understand and be threatened by it.
   b. Overt activity. Need to find the therapeutically optimum bal-
      ance between the amount of patient initiative and staff
      initiative involved in establishing a relationship and main-
      taining the program. The staff will need to be more active
      with a withdrawn patient and less active with a patient who
      has to control his therapy more.
   c. Certain expectations. Refers to the extent that patient's be-
      havior will be manipulated or controlled, not to the outcomes.

Attitudes have to be defined as well as stated. There are two categories of attitudes:

1. General attitudes - some of the ones selected by the Menninger
   Clinic are: indulgence, active friendliness, kind firmness,
   watchfulness.
2. Attitudes for specific situations such as: patient's requests of
   personnel, personnel's requests of patient, handling patient's
   privileges and restrictions.

The social role of the patient is modified and more effective behavior
patterns are developed. The therapeutic milieu provides satisfying
relationships, reduces intrapsychic conflicts, and strengthens the
ego functions.

New behavior patterns can be reinforced by providing opportunities
for the patient to practice them and by explaining the reality of his
behavior to him.

Whether on an inpatient unit in a public, private, or state hospital,
the nurse is involved with a caste system, sick patients and varying
degrees of rigidity and control, and 24 hour-a-day nursing care for
the patient.

In partial hospitalization (day, night, evening or weekend), the patients are able to function at least at times; the structure is less
rigid and the 24 hours of care have to be truncated into six. The
nurse will become more flexible, perceptive, and realistic as she
works in the "immediate" situation.

Outpatient facilities are the most unstructured and may offer crisis intervention, treatments, and psychotherapy, and focus upon taking help to the community rather than bringing the community to them. The patient seeks help on his own and is more amenable to therapy.

Although community support for mental health centers has not been overwhelming, more consideration is being given to them. The community may view sexual deviants, drug addicts, and alcoholics as unpopular and unchangeable, but the community has also supported community centers to handle crises of attempted suicide, rape, deviation, adolescent drug addicts and has not stopped supporting them.

The government has consistently supported Mental Health Centers with money and laws. They are still the most prolific researchers into mental health and mental illness. Mental health laws are constantly being reappraised and rewritten at state level.

REVIEW QUESTIONS

1. What services are the Community Mental Health Centers supposed to provide to the community?
2. Why are some patients hospitalized while others are not?
3. How do day, night, and evening hospitals differ?
4. What is a therapeutic community?
5. What are some of the advantages of ward meetings in public hospitals?
6. How does the psychiatric team function now? What were the various roles in the older team?
7. How can change be instituted in a state mental hospital?
8. What is the primary focus of outpatient clinics?

SUGGESTED REFERENCES

1. Astrachan, B., et al.: Systems approach to day hospitalization, Arch Gen Psychi XXII:550-559, 1970

2. Feder, S.: The indications and techniques of partial hospitalization, Current Psychiatric Therapies, Grune & Stratton, New York, pp. 167-174, 1971

3. Feirstein, A., et al.: A crisis intervention model for inpatient hospitalization, Current Psychiatric Therapies, Masserman, J., Ed., Grune & Stratton, New York, pp. 183-190, 1971

4. Fried, S.R., et al.: Partial hospitalization services in a private sector community mental health consortium, International J Social Psychi XIX:91-101, 1973

5. Hanson, E.T.: Nurse practitioners in ambulatory psychiatric care, Nursing Clinics N Am, W.B. Saunders Co., Philadelphia, Vol. VIII, pp. 313-323, 1973

6. Holmes, M. and Werner, J.: Psychiatric Nursing in a Therapeutic Community, The Macmillan Co., New York, 1966

7. Lynch, C.: Management of nursing care on a psychiatric service, Nursing Clinics N Am, W.B. Saunders Co., Philadelphia, Vol. VIII, pp. 293-303, 1973

8. Smiley, C.W.: The advocacy program, Perspectives Psychi Care X:220-225, 1972

9. Swartzburg, M. and Schwartz, A.: A five-year study of brief hospitalization, Am J Psychi CXXXIII:922-924, 1976

10. Tannenbaum, G.: The walk-in clinic, American Handbook of Psychiatry, Arieti, S., Ed., Basic Books, Inc., New York, Vol. III, pp. 577-587, 1966

11. Wahl, C.W.: The technique of brief psychotherapy with hospitalized psychosomatic patients, International J Psychoanalytic Psychother I:69-82, 1972

12. Zwerling, I.: Aftercare systems, American Handbook of Psychiatry, Arieti, S., Ed., Basic Books, New York, Vol. V, pp. 721-736, 1975

CHAPTER 20

SOMATIC THERAPIES

ELECTROSHOCK THERAPY

Electroconvulsive therapy (ECT) was introduced by Cerletti and Bini in 1937 and their technique is still used, with alternating current and voltage between 70 and 150 volts applied for 0.1 to 1.0 second to induce a 45-second grand mal convulsion.

There are no known contraindications for ECT but certain medicolegal precautions are taken such a general physical, electrocardiogram, and lateral x-rays of the spine.

ECT may be given in hospitals, clinics, or the doctor's office. The nurse is involved in all aspects of ECT. Primarily she provides physical care before and after and provides support and communication throughout.

Preparation (may vary in different localities: no breakfast, leave bridgework in, etc.).

1. To minimize the possibility of nausea, vomiting, or voiding after the seizure, limit intake to a light breakfast at least two hours before treatment and have patient void.
2. Remove jewelry, hairpins, and other metal objects to prevent breakage and possible injury.
3. Remove dentures to avoid injury during convulsion.
4. Have patient wear pajamas if hospitalized, or remove any tight clothes if an outpatient, loosen belts, collars, ties, to prevent interference with respirations and circulation.
5. Check the chart for all lab data and treatment permits; give any medications ordered (succinylcholine as muscle relaxant); check machine; position the patient (in whatever position used in the institution; this varies); apply electrodes to patient's head.

During convulsive treatment (opinions differ on whether to press on chin or on jaw, whether to restrain or not to restrain).

1. Mouth gag is inserted and gentle pressure is exerted on the chin.
2. Arms are folded across the chest and gentle pressure exerted on shoulders and thighs to prevent fractures of long bones and vertebrae.

Post-treatment

1. Check for respiratory difficulties, give artificial respiration if necessary until effects of muscle-relaxant wear off.

2. Observe for any signs of fracture - most common being compression fractures of the spine.
3. Put up bedrails until he is completely reacted and not excited or combative.
4. Reassure him that blurred vision, confusion, and loss of memory are temporary.
5. Help him recall events and knowledge that are important to him.
6. Support the patient if impotence or cessation of menstruation occur.

There is no simple, accepted explanation for the effectiveness of ECT. Some theorists stress the somatic effects of the convulsion itself, others stress the psychological effects of the patient's seeing ECT as a punishment.

Today ECT is used primarily with depressed patients, whether they are psychotic, senile, or involutional, and sometimes it is used with schizophrenic patients and the suicidal. There are some theories that repeated treatments may result in permanent brain damage (Templer).

Alexander and Berkeley found ECT to be most effective in treating psychotic and borderline patients whose depressions involved loss with guilt. ECT was least effective in neurotic depressions involving the basic issue of power or its loss.

Some general statements about ECT can be made:

1. It is most effective in dealing with acute, short-term illnesses.
2. It modifies symptoms but does not result in long-term improvement.
3. It is more effective when used in conjunction with other therapies.

DRUG THERAPY

During the last 20 years, the advent of drug therapy changed psychiatric treatment more than any other single development.

Acute psychotic patients were able to function without restraints, hydrotherapy, ECT. They could have their doors unlocked and be free to move about.

However, the problems of drug addiction and drug dependence have caused a closer scrutiny of drug therapy. There is some concern about the example that such reliance on drugs sets for the youth of the country.

The psychiatric nurse is responsible for establishing and maintaining the patient's drug therapy. She needs to know the expected effects and the side effects of the drugs she gives. She needs to know usual dosages to avoid errors. Once a specific drug is ordered, the nurse:

1. Administers the drug
2. Observes the effects

3. Evaluates the effects
4. Records both untoward and expected effects

The attitude of the medicine "giver" influences the effects of the medicine. Anyone can convince, consciously or otherwise, that he expects a drug to be efficacious or that he really thinks it's a waste of time to take it.

In psychiatry, especially, the nurse needs to have an effective "drug" attitude and to be aware of what her behavior is saying to the patient. She needs to understand behavior and body language, to use a variety of techniques with different patients or in different situations, and to be certain patients do not hoard drugs instead of taking them.

Psychiatric drugs are groups of specific drugs which have specific purposes and actions. The patient's symptoms, rather than his diagnosis, determine which drug will be most effective. The psychiatrist's individual preferences also influence the choice of a specific drug.

Psychiatric drugs are considered to be tranquilizing or nontranquilizing. Tranquilizing drugs may be classified as major (antipsychotic) or minor (antianxiety). The nontranquilizing drugs are also classified as antidepressants.

ANTIPSYCHOTIC AGENTS: Chemically, there are four major groups of antipsychotic drugs:

1. Phenothiazines
2. Rauwolfia alkaloids
3. Thioxanthenes
4. Butyrophenones

The rauwolfia alkaloids are not used as much as phenothiazines because they are slower-acting and may have side effects that the phenothiazines do not, such as depression or gastrointestinal hemorrhage. They are cheaper, however, and in many state hospitals are used even when other antipsychotic drugs would be preferred.

ANTIPSYCHOTIC AGENTS

	Generic Name	Trade Name
Phenothiazines	Chlorpromazine	Thorazine
	Promazine	Sparine
	Triflupromazine	Vesprin
	Thioridazine	Mellaril
	Trifluoperazine	Stelazine
	Perphenazine	Trilafon
	Prochlorperazine	Compazine
	Fluphenazine	Prolixin

Rauwolfia Alkaloids	Reserpine	Serpasil
Thioxanthenes	Chlorprothixene	Taractin
	Thiothixene	Navane
Butyrophenones	Haloperidol	Haldol

Phenothiazines are effective in treating the excited, assaultive patient who needs rapid sedation, and also the withdrawn and apathetic patient.

The more bizarre the behavior, the more quickly changes will be noted. Usually mood stabilization and more regular habit patterns are established within six weeks. Patients who have been discharged on maintenance doses may be able to continue functioning effectively for five years or more.

Individual phenothiazines may differ in effectiveness and in reactions but there are common side effects:

1. Extrapyramidal
   a. Parkinsonism - unsteady gait, hand tremor, drooling, muscular rigidity.
   b. Dyskinesia - rhythmic stereotyped motions such as lisping movements of tongue and mouth, pacing.
   c. Dystonia - severe torticollis or opisthotonos. Difficulty swallowing or opening mouth.
2. Eye and skin
   a. Blurred vision - corneal opacities, sometimes cataracts, pigmentary changes in conjunctivae with a brown discoloration, possibly acute myopia, photosensitivity.
   b. Allergic skin reactions - (nurse may also develop contact dermatitis when giving Thorazine injections or concentrate) changes in skin pigment with a bluish tint developing over areas exposed to sunlight.
3. Autonomic disturbances - Nasal congestion, dry mouth, pupil contraction, headaches, leg pain, constipation, diarrhea, impotence, menstrual irregularities, galactorrhea, breast enlargement, hypotension, weight gain.

Any of the phenothiazines can produce hypoglycemia and trigger diabetes in latent or prediabetic individuals.

All the phenothiazines have antiemetic actions, can mask serious conditions that are accompanied by nausea or vomiting.

In addition to the above effects, there are serious but more rare complications:

1. Jaundice - usually self-limited, but signs of jaundice may be indication to discontinue the drug.
2. Agranulocytosis - occurs between third and tenth weeks of therapy. Indications are: sore throat, elevated temperature, lesions or ulcerations in the mouth, infection. The condition

develops rapidly and if the acute phase is not fatal, the blood count returns to normal within a week.
3. Convulsions.

Rauwolfia alkaloids are effective in the treatment of hyperactive children, senility, acute and chronic schizophrenia, especially helpful with agitated, hypertensive, unmanageable patients.

Reserpine is slower acting than the phenothiazines and may cause drastic drop in blood pressure. Parkinsonism may be severe; any of the other phenothiazine side effects may occur.

Chlorprothixene has a clinical effect similar to Thorazine and seems to have both stimulating and relaxing actions. It produces fewer side effects related to liver, eyes, or blood but Parkinsonism is present.

Haloperidol has a completely different chemical structure than the other antipsychotic drugs. It is less sedating than the others, but has a calming effect; however, it produces more extrapyramidal effects than the others.

The antipsychotic drugs potentiate the action of certain other drugs such as:

1. Antihypertensives
2. Barbiturates
3. Alcohol
4. Narcotics

Patients should be observed for serious hypotension or depressed central nervous system reactions. Patients need to be cautioned not to combine tranquilizers and alcohol in particular since this is not an unusual practice.

These drugs interfere with coordination and motor skills. Patients need to be cautioned about driving, working with machinery, or attempting activities that are dangerous when coordination is poor.

Antipsychotic drugs may also produce extreme depression and the patient may become worse rather than better. The patient may also become more irritable or agitated, may hallucinate.

ANTIANXIETY AGENTS: The antianxiety drugs are effective in controlling mild symptoms of anxiety, the hyperexcitability of alcoholism, and in some depressions.

Some of the "mild tranquilizers" have antihistamine or muscle relaxant actions.

202 / Somatic Therapies

ANTIANXIETY AGENTS

	Generic Name	Trade Name
Benzodiazepines	Chlordiazepoxide	Librium
	Diazepam	Valium
Glycols	Meprobamate	Equanil, Miltown
Diphenylmethanes	Hydroxyzine	Atarax, Vistaril
	Azacylonol	Frenquel

Little is known about the antianxiety agents beyond the facts
that they:

1. Can lead to habituation
2. Can lead to addiction with specific withdrawal symptoms
3. Potentiate the effects of alcohol

Their most common side effects are:

1. Drowsiness
2. Ataxia

Librium and Valium are used by millions of Americans. They are
effective in treating the tense, anxious, and agitated, as well as
alcoholics and the hypoactive. Valium may reduce hostility;
Librium has little effect here.

Meprobamate was the first antianxiety drug and dates from the early
fifties. Just saying "Miltown" was enough to cause gales of laughter
on TV comedy shows of that day. This drug is addictive and has
been known to cause withdrawal symptoms including convulsions.

Atarax is characteristic of the diphenylmethane group. It is effect-
tive in treating patients with organic problems whose apprehension
interferes with healing and rest.

Because the antianxiety agents are so often prescribed for "normal"
people with milder anxiety problems, there are inherent dangers.

Mixing tranquilizers and alcohol is a common practice among the
American middle-class. This past-time has become a matter of
some concern. Tranquilizers potentiate the effects of alcohol and
can result in death.

Are all the drugs prescribed necessary? Are the drugs a "mass
crutch"? Problems have to be faced only when they are irritating.
When drugs can make one impervious to the irritation, the problems
"go away" and don't have to be faced.

Are the drugs influential in private drug addiction? Do children
"pop pills" because they see it done at home - without regard for
value or effect?

Are drugs just a "cop-out"? Are they prescribed to avoid having to bother with a patient's problem?

The antianxiety drugs are being re-evaluated by society and by medicine. Often nothing is gained by their use. Sometimes they are combined with other "perk-up" drugs to maintain a balance of tension needed to function.

It is difficult to assess the value of antianxiety drugs. Yet, of the top 200 drugs (new and refill prescriptions) for the last five years, Valium and Librium have ranked in the first five, with Valium consistently ranked number one.

ANTIDEPRESSANT AGENTS: Once the agitated excited patient had been helped with tranquilizers, the search was on for a drug that could elevate the mood of the depressed patient. Amphetamines had been used as stimulants but they had serious side effects.

One of the first antidepressives was Imipramine (Tofranil) dating from the late fifties. Many more antidepressant drugs have been developed since then and have yet to be effectively evaluated.

ANTIDEPRESSANT AGENTS

	Generic Name	Trade Name
Tricyclics	Imipramine	Tofranil
	Amitriptyline	Elavil
	Nortriptyline	Aventyl
	Doxepin	Sinequan
MAO Inhibitors	Isocarboxazid	Marplan
	Phenelzine	Nardil
	Tranylcypromine	Parnate
Psychomotor Stimulants	Amphetamine	Benzedrine
	Dextroamphetamine	Dexedrine
	Methamphetamine	Methedrine
	Methylphenidate	Ritalin

Every type of antidepressant drug has had its problems. One of the first - Iproniazid (Marsilid) - was taken off the market because of its severe side effects. Monoamine Oxidase inhibitors are toxic, potent, have serious side effects and many of them have been removed from the market. Amphetamines have been re-evaluated in the light of recent increases in drug addiction and were removed from the market in 1973.

Any antidepressant may mask the symptoms of a potential suicide and close observation is necessary to prevent suicidal actions.

Tofranil produces a gradual mood elevation in both exogenous and endogenous depressions. Elavil is considered more effective in endogenous depressions. Aventyl is effective in treating the acute panic states in phobias.

The side effects of the tricyclics are many but generally reversible if detected early. Some of the less serious side effects are:

1. Autonomic disturbances - dry mouth, blurred vision, constipation, dizziness, vomiting, sweating (especially about the head and neck), hypotension, urinary retention, impotence.
2. Allergic reactions.
3. Fine tremors (sometimes of the tongue).
4. Visual hallucinations, hypotonic excitement, insomnia.
5. Withdrawal symptoms - nausea, vomiting, headache, chills, cold sweat, insomnia, abdominal cramps, anxiety, diarrhea.

Two of the most serious side effects are:

1. Acute congestive glaucoma in predisposed patients and aggravation of glaucoma, if present.
2. Cardiovascular complications including congestive heart failure, coronary thrombosis and EKG changes, especially in the elderly.

MAO inhibitors are potent but relatively unsafe. Nardil is considered the most toxic; Parnate was withdrawn from the market temporarily because of its side effects.

They are probably no more effective in treating depressions than the tricyclics, are far more dangerous, and slower-acting. They have some success in treating phobias.

Some of the minor side effects are: dry mouth, dizziness, orthostatic hypotension, urinary problems, delayed ejaculation, impotence, confusion, disorientation. The more serious side effects can be fatal:

1. Liver damage, hepatitis similar to viral hepatitis, necrosis of the liver.
2. Hypertensive crisis
   a. Headaches with high blood pressure, chills, stiff neck, nausea and vomiting, sweating, twitching.
   b. Severe hypertension with chest pains, apprehension, diaphoresis, collapse.
   c. Cerebral hemorrhage with chest pains, palpitations, high blood pressure, sweating and pallor.

Hypertensive crisis is directly related to drugs and diet. MAO inhibitors taken in conjunction with such drugs as tricyclics or amphetamines can be fatal. When changing medications from an MAO to a tricyclic or the reverse, the patient should have at least two weeks between without medicine.

Severe hypertensive crises resulting in death have been precipitated by eating foods containing large amounts of Tyramine, an amine usually destroyed by MAO. Such foods include:

1. Aged cheese, especially cheddar, limburger, gouda, Stilton.
2. Chianti wine and beer.
3. Chicken livers and pickled herring.
4. Broad beans and yeast products.
5. Chocolate.

Such crises have occurred within two to twenty hours after eating cheese.

The stimulants were the first drugs used in treating depression. They act directly on the nervous system, fast-acting but wear off quickly. When they wear off in three to four hours, a worse slump results.

Many drug addicts take them for kicks and they do give a sense of euphoria, well-being, alertness, and energy. They are prescribed as mood elevators, appetite depressants, or to counteract hyperactivity in children.

Some of the lesser side effects:

1. Agitation, combativeness.
2. Insomnia.
3. Inability to concentrate.
4. Decreased appetite.
5. Decreased sexual desire and some degree of impotency.
6. Hypomania.

Among the most serious side effects are:

1. Increased suicide risk as "let-down" brings deeper depression.
2. Psychotic-like paranoid reactions with hallucinations, delusions.
3. Early tolerance requiring larger doses.
4. Addiction with withdrawal symptoms.

The addictive problems and psychotic reactions are two effects which led to the removal of amphetamines from the market.

OTHER PSYCHIATRIC DRUGS

Lithium Carbonate (Lithium)

Long used in Australia and Europe for treating manic states, lithium has recently been introduced to the United States. It is considered by many to be the drug of choice in the treatment of mania. Some feel that it not only produces a remission of symptoms but actually prevents a recurrence of the manic state.

There must be a certain blood level of lithium obtained before it is effective. This may take up to 10 days. The patient on lithium is happy and feels excited without manic elation. The exact mechanism of action is as yet unknown.

Some side effects are: nausea, vomiting, diarrhea, thirst, muscle weakness, tinnitus, vertigo, blurred vision, confusion.

When salt intake is not maintained or side effects ignored, patients may develop lithium intoxication symptoms:

1. Excessive thirst
2. Polyuria
3. Ataxia
4. Persistent diarrhea and vomiting
5. Nystagmus
6. Seizures
7. Anuria
8. Coma

Sodium depletion may also occur in hot weather or during exercise or activities that cause excessive perspiration. Crash diets have the same effect and fasting sprees must be avoided. Since manic patients do not attend to their physical ailments, close observation is necessary to monitor possible toxic effects. Patients need to be cautioned not to change the dosage, increasing the dose does not increase the effectiveness but it does increase the toxicity.

Disulfiram (Antabuse)

Introduced in the late forties to "cure" alcoholics, Antabuse is an unpleasant drug and has had poor results.

The drug has no effect until alcohol is consumed; then the reactions experienced are assumed to deter further consumption of alcohol. It remains effective in the body for several days but need only be stopped if the alcoholic wishes to resume drinking. When implanted surgically, the period of abstinence has been longer (Malcolm).

When alcohol reacts with Antabuse the patient experiences:

1. Extreme nausea and vomiting
2. Throbbing headache
3. Palpitations and dyspnea
4. Blurred vision

To be effective, Antabuse needs to be reinforced with psychotherapy.

Antiparkinsonism Agents

Used to counteract the "Parkinsonism" side effects of the antipsychotic drugs:

1. Trihexphenidyl (Artane)
2. Benztropine Methanesulfonate (Cogentin)
3. Procyclidine (Kemadrin)

All are muscle relaxants that reduce rigidity and tremors. Secretion of saliva is diminished and reflex swallowing facilitated. Side effects are few: dry mouth, drowsiness, blurred vision, dizziness.

The nurse who administers psychiatric drugs has to be observant for the drugs may mask dangerous symptoms (suicidal impulses) and it is sometimes difficult to differentiate side effects from symptoms.

For instance, impotence may be a symptom of depression and also a side effect of antidepressant drugs. The patient may be less "agitated" if he knows such a side effect exists and that it is temporary.

As with any other medications, the nurse is responsible for knowing the dosage, actions, and side effects of the drugs as well as for administering them as prescribed.

She needs to observe the patient for evidence of drug action, to question him and be sure that he is feeling the way she "thinks" he's feeling.

Drugs may mask problems and the nurse, being in close contact with the patient, is in a position to obtain relevant information for intervention.

RESTITUTIVE THERAPY

The various techniques used to produce altered states of consciousness have been known for centuries. Thousands of years ago alcohol, mescaline and sacred mushrooms were used in religious ceremonies and as curatives.

LSD (lysergic acid diethylamide) was discovered accidentally in 1943 and was later used to induce "model psychoses" as an aid in insight therapy. In large doses, LSD can produce an intense transcendental experience. Much research was done with LSD in the fifties. Marijuana, known in Asia for more than 5000 years, became the favorite psychoactive drug of the youth culture during the sixties. It remains almost as controversial today as it was in 1965.

In the seventies, transcendental meditation replaced the LSD experience as the ultimate road to self-awareness. Biofeedback came into vogue as a way to demonstrate the power of mind over body in controlling the alpha wave activity.

The nurse may be involved with altered states of consciousness in patients' therapy or as she pursues her own transcendental experiences.

Pahnke described the nine interrelated categories derived from content-analysis of mystical consciousness experiences.

1. Unity may be internal or external
   a. Internal unity refers to the transcending of self and the inner world within the experiencer. Sense impressions cease and the individuality or the ego fades away. Consciousness of what is being experienced expands and the experiencer has

a sense of relinquishing life, of approaching reality, of life and death as one.

b. External unity refers to the transcending of self and the external world outside the experience. One or more sense impression grows in intensity until the subject and the object cease to exist as separate entities. The object may be a rose, a book, a grain of sand, a note of music - but ultimately the experiencer becomes One with the object and has the insight that "we are all the same thing".

2. Objectivity and Reality involve insightful knowledge about existence or being on a nonrational or intuitive level gained by direct experience and the certainty that the knowledge is real whereas the experience may be felt to be subjective or delusional. One answers the question of "what am I?" or may experience the great brotherhood of man.

3. Transcendance of Time and Space refers to the loss of orientation in the usual three-dimensional perception of environment and suddenly feeling outside of time and space. One experiences the unbroken continuity of past, present and future.

4. Sense of Sacredness is a feeling of awe or reverence or holiness more basic than the experiencer's religious concepts, a feeling of humility in the presence of the Infinite.

5. Deeply-felt Positive Mood may range from an intense spiritual sexual orgasm to the deep relaxation of the "peace which passes all understanding".

6. Paradoxicality reflects the claims that violate the laws of logic such as "out of the body" experiences while still in the body.

7. Alleged Ineffability makes communication of experiences impossible for there are no words to describe them adequately.

8. Transiency refers to the temporary duration of the experience compared to the relative permanence of usual experiences. Transiency is one of the important differences between the mystical state and psychosis.

9. Positive Changes in Attitude or Behavior are reported by those experiencing the preceding eight categories. They feel a greater sense of self-worth, increased personal integration, greater sensitivity to the eternals and loss of fear of death as well as an expanded awareness of existence and of creation.

Not all altered states of consciousness are mystical. There are nonmystical experiences of an esthetic, psychodynamic, psychotic or cognitive nature identified by Pahnke.

1. Aesthetic phenomena include changes in spatial perception. Distances are altered, colors may be brighter, objects may become distorted. The experiencer may feel his body is melting away or fragmenting.

2. Psychodynamic phenomena occur as a regression to early childhood or to infancy and the re-experiencing of traumatic moments. Guilt may be faced or grief or hostility felt with great intensity. These experiences can be therapeutic if professional help is available when they occur. Without supervision, some of these experiences can lead to decompensation.

3. Psychotic phenomena manifest as paranoia or panic with confusion and disorientation. One can "go in" and "come out" of the
   experiences almost at will.
4. Cognitive phenomena involve the process of thinking rather than
   of intuition. Associations and inferences occur in rapid succes-
   sion and one is aware of ideas and their inter-relationships.

Other phenomena do not fit into any of the categories: seeing bright
white lights, feeling the flow of electrical energy in the body, tele-
pathic or clairvoyant experiences, changes in perception of time
and increased awareness of somatic changes.

LSD, MEDITATION AND BIOFEEDBACK: One of the most potent
drugs known to man, LSD is the most familiar of the psychodelic
or mind expanding drugs. It has been used in Great Britain and
Canada in treatment of alcoholic patients and experimentally in the
United States with autism and with the terminally ill. In small frequent doses, LSD is considered to be useful in making the patient
more open to therapy, especially those patients who use repression
or denial as their primary defense mechanism. One large single
dose supposedly will facilitate a reintegration of the personality by
producing the psychodynamic phenomenon of regression to infancy
or childhood.

However, LSD has not proven to be an effective therapeutic drug.
Although tolerance develops rapidly and is lost rapidly, physical
dependence does not occur and psychological dependence is rare.
The effects may range from aesthetic phenomena and heightened or
distorted sensory perceptions to a powerful mystical experience to
a frank psychotic break.

The greatest risk with LSD is the possibility of precipitating such
psychotic episodes. The acute episodes (bad trips) last less than 24
hours but the chronic states may involve irreversible deterioration
and ultimately institutionalization.

There is always a danger of harm to the subject or to others as he
feels powerful enough to "fly" out of a window or paranoid enough to
attack his "enemies". A characteristic effect is the "flashback" or
spontaneous recurrence of a "trip" months after the drug was taken
and the trip occurred.

LSD affects primarily the central nervous system and the user may
have dilated pupils, tremors, increased temperature and higher
blood pressure and hyperactive reflexes. On the EEG, LSD produces increased beta wave activity, common also in delirium and
hallucinations.

Although beta wave activity is present at the beginning of meditation,
alpha wave activity rapidly increases and later theta and delta
waves. Alpha waves are present in alert, waking states and theta
and delta in sleep. Transcendental meditation (TM) is a relaxing
way to achieve an altered state of consciousness, usually of the mystical type. Once LSD users become successful meditators, they are

not as likely to use drugs to "trip". If they discontinue meditation, however, they may return to LSD.

Physiologically meditation decreases blood pressure and muscle activity and increases skin resistance. The body is relaxed, yet the mind is alert and able to control physiological responses.

The hallmark of TM is the use of a personal mantra. A mantra is a sound that is life supporting to the individual. Each person has a private mantra. Thinking or silently repeating one's mantra has a powerful effect on the central nervous system, promoting ease and order in brain wave activity and relaxation of the body. TM is a permissive and entirely intrapersonal technique, sometimes more effective than drugs for inducing relaxation and lessening anxiety in patients.

Personality changes occur in patients who meditate regularly. Increased energy and less tension decrease anxiety and improve physical stamina and creative activity. Meditation fosters a sense of self that is sometimes threatening to those who are used to playing the self-effacing role. The affective changes that leave the individual thoughtful and in touch with his feelings provide a post-meditative period which is fruitful for psychotherapy sessions.

Meditation may produce changes that are not compatible with the pathological life style. Unless the resistance is dealt with, meditation may be abandoned in the interest of maintaining psychic or emotional comfort. Insight into the resistance is necessary for successful psychotherapy with meditation.

In meditation, the physiological processes may be deliberately controlled and altered by the meditative process itself. Biofeedback is a scientific way to control processes that are normally not within conscious awareness by using a combination of meditation and technology. The biofeedback machine is an EEG that reinforces alpha wave responses. The subject, attached to the machine, performs meditative and other autogenic exercises. When an exercise has the desired effect on brain wave activity, the machine signals. With practice the reinforced effect can be produced at will. Specific exercises can be repeated until the heart rate, stomach acid, blood pressure, etc. can be controlled. Biofeedback has been used to produce altered states of consciousness. It can be used to facilitate creative activity, to induce relaxation and has been most successful in treating patients manifesting psychosomatic symptoms.

Recently other somatic therapies have appeared including:

(1) structured integration (Rolfing) which focuses on deep muscle manipulation using elbows as well as hands as a means of decreasing muscular rigidity, releasing emotions and restructuring the body into natural alignment with gravitational forces; (2) Silva mind control that relies on a self-hypnosis and meditation approach in which the subject "visualizes" solutions to his problems; and (3) the Fieldenkraus method that reverses the usual mind-body relationship and teaches that by changing body movements (with some 30,000 exer-

cises) one can change thinking and feeling patterns, even reversing the aging process and relieving such nervous system diseases as multiple sclerosis.

Only the future practitioners can decide whether these various mind altering practices are effective personally or useful therapeutically.

REVIEW QUESTIONS

1. For what condition is ECT most often used?
2. How is a patient prepared for ECT?
3. What does the post-convulsive care include?
4. What are the major classifications of psychiatric drugs? How do they differ?
5. What does a nurse do once a drug has been ordered?
6. For what does a nurse observe after administering a medication?
7. What are some of the side effects of Thorazine? Librium? Tofranil?
8. What are the dangers of MAO inhibitors?
9. What foods should be avoided when taking MAO inhibitors?
10. If a patient's drug is changed from Tofranil (last dose Monday P.M.) to Parnate (first dose Tuesday A.M.) what should the nurse know? What should she do?
11. What are the disadvantages of amphetamines?
12. For what condition is lithium recommended?
13. What is disulfiram? How is it used?
14. What drugs are helpful to counteract the extrapyramidal effects of antipsychotic drugs?
15. What is an altered state of consciousness?
16. How can LSD be used most effectively?
17. What are the uses of meditation and biofeedback?

SUGGESTED REFERENCES

1. Alexander, L., et al.: Which antidepressant for which patient? Med Insight, pp. 12-19, Feb., 1972

2. Bergerson, B.S.: Pharmacology in Nursing, C.V. Mosby, St. Louis, 1973

3. Bloomfield, H.H. and Kory, R.B.: Happiness, the TM Program, Psychiatry, and Enlightenment, Simon & Schuster, New York, 1976

4. Carrington, P. and Harmon, S.E.: Clinical use of meditation in Current Psychi Therapies XV:101-108, 1975

5. Clower, C.G.: Convulsive therapy, Medical Counterpoint, pp. 31-311, Feb., 1970

6. Fieve, R.R., et al.: Lithium prophylaxis of depression in Bipolar I, Bipolar II, and Unipolar patients, Am J Psychi CXXXIII:925-939, 1976

7. Fink, M., et al.: Narcotic antagonists: Another approach to addiction therapy, Am J Nursing CXXI:1350-1368, July, 1971

8. Glueck, B. and Stroebel, C.F.: Biofeedback and meditation in the treatment of psychiatric illness, Current Psychi Therapies XV:109-118, 1975

9. Goodman, L.S. and Gilman, A.: The Pharmacological Basis of Therapeutics, Macmillan, New York, 1970

10. Goth, A.: Medical Pharmacology, C.V. Mosby, St. Louis, 1974

11. Govoni, L.E. and Hayes, J.E.: Drugs and Nursing Implications, 2nd Ed., Appleton-Century-Crofts, New York, 1971

12. Hollister, L.E.: Uses of psychotropic drugs, Ann Intern Med LXXIX:88-98, 1973

13. Kline, N. and Davis, J.M.: Psychotropic drugs, Am J Nursing LXXIII:54-62, 1973

14. Lawrence, J.: Alpha Brain Waves, Avon, New York, 1972

15. Ludwig, A.M. and Surawicz, F.G.: Restitutive therapies, In American Handbook of Psychiatry, 2nd Ed., Arieti, S., Ed., Vol. V, pp. 514-524, 1975

16. Malcolm, M.T. and Madden, J.S.: The use of disulfiram implantation in alcoholism, Br J Psychi CXXIII:41-45, July, 1973

17. Mendels, J.: Lithium in the treatment of depression, Am J Psychi CXXXIII:373-378, 1976

18. Pahnke, W.N. and Richards, W.A.: Implications of LSD and experimental mysticism, J Religion Health V:175-208, 1966

19. Rosenthal, S.H.: Alterations in serum thyroxine with cerebral therapy, Arch Gen Psychi XXVIII:28-29, 1973

20. Shevitz, S.A.: Psychosurgery: Some current observations, Am J Psychi CXVXIII:37-40, 1976

21. Stroebel, C. and Glueck, B.: Biofeedback treatment in medicine and psychiatry: An ultimate placebo? Seminars Psychi V:379-393, 1973

22. Swonger, A.K. and Constantine, L.L.: Drugs and Therapy, Little, Brown & Co., Inc., Boston, 1976

23. Tart, C., Ed.: Altered States of Consciousness, John Wiley & Sons, Inc., New York, 1969

24. Templer, D.I., et al.: Cognitive functioning and degree of psychosis in schizophrenics given many electro-convulsive treatments, Br J Psychi CXXIII:441-443, Sept., 1973

CRITERIA FOR RATING SUICIDAL INTENTION*
(Assessment of the wish to destroy oneself)

A. ADEQUACY OF PLANNING

Description:

No planning, no preparation apparent. Can include acknowledgment that "S" thought about suicide or death, but with no action on them.

Intent inferred by actions, but otherwise ambiguous with no planning in preparation, or information. The observed suicidal behavior is impulsive, psychotic or intoxicated, and includes accidental features like falling, breaking structures, lack of judgment.

Implicit intent apparent by prior threats or verbalizations. Planning is superficial; has knowledge of a method or place demonstrated by actual attempt. Opportunistic features prominent (e.g., suicidal behavior noted only with alcohol ingestion, but no information otherwise).

Explicit intent apparent. Some preparation in evidence (e.g., efforts to accumulate pills or obtain guns, but no setting of time or place).

Explicit intent apparent. Advanced preparation with respect to availability of method, and either place or time; not both (or no information). Shorter interval between first effort and attempt behavior.

Explicit intent apparent. Advanced preparation with respect to availability of method, and either place or time; not both (or no information). Shorter interval between first effort and attempt behavior.

Explicit intent apparent. Advanced preparation with respect to availability of method, place, and time; "alcohol for courage". Longer interval between first effort and attempt behavior.

Explicit intent apparent. Same as #5 above but with evidence of knowledgeability with respect to method, place, and movements of potential rescuers (e.g., notes prepared beforehand, wills, alcohol/pills by a physician or pharmacist, etc.). Exclude impulsive behavior, CO poisoning.

B. EFFECTIVENESS OF METHOD (lethality)

Method Description:

Self-injury simulating, but no damage possible (e.g., threatens self with toy gun, or drinks colored water claiming it to be poison).

* Dr. F. Cutter of the Los Angeles Suicide Prevention Clinic, prepared this scale. Scores range from 0 to 18.

Inadequate or ineffectual methods (e.g., swallowed buttons, overdose of castor oil as youth or adult, swallowed cloth and toothbrush).

Low order of effectiveness (e.g., scratch or superficial cutting of own wrist to unspecified depth, banged on walls, or pushed hand through glass window).

Low, moderate effectiveness (e.g., deep cut on wrist requires sutures; jumped or waded into shallow water; ingested nonprescription pills, e.g., aspirin, sleeping tablets, or small and/or unknown amounts of pills; ate four toadstools).

Ambiguous outcomes (e.g., ingested prescription pills (with alcohol) but amount unknown; cut tendons and vein in wrist or elbow; stabbing; turned on gas in room; jumped in front of or out of an automobile; jumped off pier into ocean; drowning; no information).

Moderate/high effectiveness (e.g., CO gas in car, cutting or stabbing of the body, injury explicit; took chloroform or other similar modes of self-asphyxiation; ingested poison, Drano, Clorox, 20 or more mixed pills, paraldehyde, carbolic acid, rat poison, etc.).

High order of effectiveness, irreversible lethal method, no time for rescue (e.g., gunshot to head, chest, abdomen; hanged self, jumped from high place, injected poisonous substance by hypodermic; jumped in front of train or truck).

C. PROVISION FOR RESCUE

Description:

Patient rescues self after an attempt, or changes mind before completing attempt.

Makes the attempt in the presence of one or more others, even with minimal or ineffectual efforts to prevent him (exclude suicide pact with significant other).

Somebody notified or sought out at the time or immediately after the attempt, especially a medical resource following ingestion method.

Somebody expected momentarily or at a definite time. "S" is counting on someone finding him and unpredictability of others could result in death.

Neither facilitates nor prevents rescue. No information. Leaves rescue to chance.

Method carried out in place where possibility of intervention is absent or minimal. Also includes significant other trying to prevent (e.g., bolts in front of vehicle in presence of others, or gunshot and jumping in presence of others). "S" made no rescue provisions himself. If he is rescued it is due to the efforts of others.

"S" takes active measures to avoid intervention, so that he cannot be found or stopped (e.g., goes to isolated place or registers in a hotel room under an assumed name).

APPENDIX B

DEVELOPMENTAL SCHEMA CHART*

THE NEWBORN AND YOUNG INFANT
(Birth to 6 Months)

Tasks in Process

INFANT

To adjust physiologically to extra-uterine life.

To develop appropriate psychologic response.

To assimilate experimentally, with increasing capacity to postpone and accept substitutes.

MOTHER

To sustain baby and self physically and pleasurably.

To give and get emotional gratification from nurturing baby.

To foster and integrate baby's development.

Acceptable Behavioral Characteristics

INFANT

Copes with mechanics of life (eating, sleeping, etc.).

Body needs urgent.

Reflexes dominate.

Has biologic unit with mother.

Establishes symbiotic relationship to mother.

Sucking behavior prominent.

Cries when distressed.

Responds to mouth, skin, sense modalities.

Is unstable physiologically.

Functions egocentrically.

MOTHER

Provides favorable feeding and handling. Gets to "know" baby.

Develops good working relationship with baby.

Has tolerance for baby.

Promotes sense of trust.

Learns baby's cues.

Applies learning to management of baby.

Interacts emotionally with baby.

Encourages baby's development.

Has reasonable expectations of baby.

* Milton, J.E. Senn and Albert J. Solnit, "Problems in Child Behavior and Development", Philadelphia: Lea & Febiger, 1968.

Is completely dependent.

Has low patience tolerance.

Is non-cognitive; expresses
needs instinctually.

Develops trust in ministering
adult.

Begins to "expect".

Minimal Psychopathology

INFANT | MOTHER

Feeding and digestive
problems.

Indifference to baby.

Sleep disturbances.

Ambivalence towards baby and
its needs.

Excessive sucking activity.

Self-doubt and anxiety.

Excessive motor discharge.

Intolerance of baby's
characteristics.

Excessive crying.

Over- or under-response to
baby.

Excessive irritability.

Hypertonicity.

Premature or inappropriate
expectations.

Difficult to comfort.

Dissatisfaction with role of
motherhood.

Extreme Psychopathology

INFANT | MOTHER

Lethargy (depression).

Alienation from baby.

Marasmus.

Severe depression.

Cannot be comforted.

Excessive guilt.

Unresponsive.

Complete inability to function
in maternal role.

Infantile autism.

Overwhelming and incapacitating
anxiety.

Developmental arrest.

Denies or tries to control baby's
needs.

Severe clashes with baby.

Vents life's dissatisfactions on baby.

(6-18 Months)
Tasks in Process

INFANT	MOTHER
To develop more reliance and self-control.	To provide a healthy emotional and physical climate.
To differentiate self from mother.	To foster weaning, training, habits.
To make developmental progress.	To understand, appreciate and accept baby.

Acceptable Behavioral Characteristics

INFANT	MOTHER
More stable physiologically.	Derives satisfaction from serving baby well.
Heightened voluntary motor activity and exploration.	Responds appropriately to baby's signs of distress.
Higher level of patience tolerance.	Aware of baby's inborn reaction pattern.
Instinctual needs in better control.	Has more confidence in own ability.
Strong selective tie to mother.	Gives positive psychologic reassurance (fondling, talking, comforting).
Stranger differentiation.	
Increased verbality, play and sensorimotor behavior.	Shows pleasure in baby.
Discernible social responses; joyful in play.	Keeps pace with baby's advances.
Outbursts of negativism and anger.	Is accepting of baby's idiosyncracies.
Sensory modalities important.	
Emergence of idiosyncratic patterns.	

Demonstrates memory and anticipation.

Begins to imitate.

Minimal Psychopathology

INFANT	MOTHER
Excessive crying, anger and irritability.	Disappointed in and unaccepting of baby.
Low frustration tolerance.	Misses baby's cues.
Excessive negativism.	Infancy unappealing.
Finicky eater, sleep disturbances.	Impersonal management.
Digestive and elimination problems.	Attempts to coerce to desired behavior.
Noticeable motility patterns (fingering, rocking, etc.).	Over-anxious or over-protective.
Delayed development.	Mildly depressed and apathetic.

Extreme Psychopathology

INFANT	MOTHER
Tantrums and convulsive disorders.	Neglect or abuse of baby.
Apathy, immobility and withdrawal.	Rejection of the maternal role.
Extreme and obsessive finger-sucking, rocking, head-banging.	Severe hostility reactions.
No interest in objects, environment or play.	No attempt to understand or gratify baby.
Anorexia.	Deliberately thwarts infant.
Megacolon.	Complete withdrawal and separation from baby.
Inexpressive of feeling.	
No social discrimination.	
No tie to mother; wary of all adults.	
Infantile autism.	

Failure to thrive.

Arrested development.

THE TODDLER AND PRE-SCHOOL AGE
(Under 5 Years)

Tasks in Process

CHILD	MOTHER
To reach physiologic plateaus (motor action, toilet training).	To promote training, habits and physiologic progression.
To differentiate self and secure sense of autonomy.	To aid in family and group socialization of child.
To tolerate separations from mother.	To encourage speech and other learning.
To develop conceptual understandings and "ethical" values.	To reinforce child's sense of autonomy and identity.
To master instinctual psychologic impulses (oedipal, sexual, guilt, shame).	To set a model for "ethical" conduct.
To assimilate and handle socialization and acculturation (aggression, relationships, activities, feelings).	To delineate male and female roles.
To learn sex distinctions.	

Acceptable Behavioral Characteristics

CHILD	MOTHER
Gratification from exercise of neuromotor skills.	Is moderate and flexible in training.
Investigative, imitative, imaginative play.	Shows pleasure and praise for child's advances.
Actions somewhat modulated by thought memory good; animistic and original thinking.	Encourages and participates with child in learning and in play.
Exercises autonomy with body (sphincter control, eating).	Sets reasonable standards and controls.
Feelings of dependence on mother and separation fears.	Paces herself to child's capacities at a given time.

Behavior identification with parents, siblings, peers.

Consistent in own behavior, conduct and ethics.

Learns speech for communication.

Provides emotional reassurance to child.

Awareness of own motives, beginnings of conscience.

Promotes peer play and guided group activity.

Intense feelings of shame, guilt, joy, love, desire to please.

Reinforces child's cognition of male and female roles.

Internalized standards of "bad", "good"; beginning of reality testing.

Broader sex curiosity and differentiation.

Ambivalence towards dependence and independence.

Questions birth and death.

Minimal Psychopathology

CHILD

MOTHER

Poor motor coordination.

Premature, coercive or censuring training.

Persistent speech problems (stammering, loss of words).

Exacting standards above child's ability to conform.

Timidity towards people and experiences.

Transmits anxiety and apprehension.

Fears and night terrors.

Unaccepting of child's efforts; intolerant towards failures.

Problems with eating, sleeping, elimination, toileting, weaning.

Over-reacts, over-protective, over-anxious.

Irritability, crying, temper tantrums.

Despondent, apathetic.

Partial return to infantile manners.

Inability to leave mother without panic.

Fear of strangers.

Breathholding spells.

Lack of interest in other children.

Extreme Psychopathology

CHILD	MOTHER
Extreme lethargy, passivity or hypermotility.	Severely coercive and punitive.
	Totally critical and rejecting.
Little or no speech; non-communicative.	Over-identification with or overly submissive to child.
No response or relationship to people, symbiotic clinging to mother.	Inability to accept child's sex; fosters opposite.
Somatic ills; vomiting, constipation, diarrhea, megacolon, rash, tics.	Substitutes child for spouse; sexual expression via child.
Autism, childhood psychosis.	Severe repression of child's need for gratification.
Excessive enuresis, soiling, fears.	Deprivation of all stimulations, freedoms and pleasures.
Completely infantile behavior.	Extreme anger and displeasure with child.
Play inhibited and non-conceptualized; absence or excess of autoerotic activity.	Child assault and brutality.
Obsessive-compulsive behavior; "ritual" bound mannerisms.	Severe depressions and withdrawal.
Impulsive destructive behavior.	

SCHOOL AGE AND PRE-ADOLESCENCE
(5 to 12 Years)

Tasks in Process

CHILD	PARENT(S)
To master greater physical prowess.	To help child's emancipation from parents.
To further establish self-identity and sex role.	To reinforce self-identification and independence.
To work towards greater independence from parents.	To provide positive pattern of social and sex role behavior.

To become aware of world-at-large.

To develop peer and other relationships.

To acquire learning, new skills and a sense of industry.

To facilitate learning, reasoning, communication and experiencing.

To promote wholesome moral and ethical values.

Acceptable Behavioral Characteristics

CHILD

General good health, greater body competence, acute sensory perception.

Pride and self-confidence; less dependence on parents.

Better impulse control.

Ambivalence re dependency, separation and new experiences.

Accepts own sex role; psychosexual expression in play and fantasy.

Equates parents with peers and other adults.

Aware of natural world (life, death, birth, science): Subjective but realistic about world.

Competitive but well organized in play; enjoys peer interaction.

Regard for collective obedience to social laws, rules and fair play.

Explores environment; school and neighborhood basic to social-learning experience.

Cognition advancing; intuitive thinking advancing to concrete operational level; responds to learning.

PARENT(S)

Ambivalent towards child's separation but encourage independence.

Mixed feelings about parent-surrogates but help child to accept them.

Encourage child to participate outside the home.

Set appropriate model of social and ethical behavior and standards.

Take pleasure in child's developing skills and abilities.

Understand and cope with child's behavior.

Find other gratifications in life (activity, employment).

Are supportive towards child as required.

Speech becomes reasoning and
expressive tool; thinking still
egocentric.

Minimal Psychopathology

CHILD

PARENT(S)

Anxiety and oversensitivity to
new experiences (school, relationships, separation).

Disinclination to separate from
child; or prematurely hastening
separation.

Lack of attentiveness; learning
difficulties, disinterest in
learning.

Signs of despondency, apathy,
hostility.

Acting out; lying, stealing, temper outbursts; inappropriate social behavior.

Foster fears, dependence,
apprehension.

Disinterested in or rejecting of
child.

Regressive behavior (wetting,
soiling, crying, fears).

Overly critical and censuring;
undermine child's confidence.

Appearance of compulsive mannerisms (tics, rituals).

Inconsistent in discipline or
control; erratic in behavior.

Somatic illness; eating and
sleeping problems, aches,
pains, digestive upsets.

Offer a restrictive, overly
moralistic model.

Fear of illness and body injury.

Difficulties and rivalry with
peers, siblings, adults; constant
fighting.

Destructive tendencies strong;
temper tantrums.

Inability or unwillingness to do
things for self.

Moodiness and withdrawal; few
friends or personal relationships.

Extreme Psychopathology

CHILD

PARENT(S)

Extreme withdrawal, apathy,
depression, grief, self-destructive tendencies.

Extreme depression and withdrawal; rejection of child.

Intense hostility; aggression
towards child.

Complete failure to learn.
Speech difficulty, especially
stuttering.

Extreme and uncontrollable antisocial behavior (aggression, destruction, chronic lying, stealing,
intentional cruelty to animals).

Severe obsessive-compulsive behavior (phobias, fantasies,
rituals).

Inability to distinguish reality
from fantasy.

Excessive sexual exhibitionism,
eroticism, sexual assaults on
others.

Extreme somatic illness: failure
to thrive, anorexia, obesity, hypochondriasis, abnormal menses.

Complete absence or deterioration of personal and peer relationships.

Uncontrollable fears, anxieties,
guilts.

Complete inability to function in
family role.

Severe moralistic prohibition of
child's independent strivings.

PUBERTY AND EARLY ADOLESCENCE
(12 to 15 Years)

Tasks in Process

CHILD

To come to terms with body
changes.

To cope with sexual development.

To establish and confirm sense
of identity.

To learn further re sex role.

To synthesize personality.

To struggle for independence
and emancipation from family.

To incorporate learning to the
gestalt of living.

PARENT(S)

To help child complete
emancipation.

To provide support and understanding.

To limit child's behavior and
set standards.

To offer favorable and appropriate environment for healthy
development.

To recall own adolescent difficulties; to accept and respect
the adolescent's differences or
similarities to parents or
others.

To relate to adolescents and
adolescence with a constructive
sense of humor.

Acceptable Behavioral Characteristics

CHILD

Heightened physical power,
strength and coordination.

Occasional psychosomatic and
somatopsychic disturbances.

Maturing sex characteristics
and proclivities.

Review and resolution of oedipal conflicts.

Inconsistent, unpredictable and
paradoxical behavior.

Exploration and experimentation with self and world.

Eagerness for peer approval
and relationships.

Strong moral and ethical perceptions.

Cognitive development accel-
erated; deductive and inductive
reasoning; operational thought.

Competitive in play; erratic
work-play patterns.

Better use of language and other
symbolic material.

Critical cf self and others; self-
evaluative.

Highly ambivalent towards
parents.

Anxiety over loss of parental
nurturing.

Hostility to parents.

Verbal aggression.

PARENT(S)

Allow and encourage reasonable
independence.

Set fair rules; are consistent.

Compassionate and understanding; firm but not punitive or
derogatory.

Feel pleasure and pride; occasional guilt and disappointment.

Have other interests besides
child.

Marital life fulfilled apart from
child.

Occasional expression of intolerance, resentment, envy or
anxiety about adolescent's
development.

Minimal Psychopathology

CHILD

Apprehensions, fears, guilt and anxiety re sex, health education.

Defiant, negative, impulsive or depressed behavior.

Frequent somatic or hypochondriacal complaints; or denial of ordinary illnesses.

Learning irregular or deficient.

Sexual preoccupation.

Poor or absent personal relationships with adults or peers.

Immaturity or precocious behavior; unchanging personality and temperament.

Unwillingness to assume the responsibility of greater autonomy.

Inability to substitute or postpone gratifications.

PARENT(S)

Sense of failure.

Disappointment greater than joy.

Indifference to child and family.

Apathy and depression.

Persistent intolerance of child.

Limited interests and self-expression.

Loss of perspective about child's capacities.

Occasional direct or vicarious reversion to adolescent impulses.

Uncertainty about standards regarding sexual behavior and deviant social or personal activity.

Extreme Psychopathology

CHILD

Complete withdrawal into self, extreme depression.

Acts of delinquency, asceticism, ritualism, over-conformity.

Neuroses, especially phobias, persistent anxiety, compulsions, inhibitions or constrictive behavior.

Persistent hypochondriases.

Sex aberrations.

Somatic illness: anorexia, colitis, menstrual disorders.

PARENT(S)

Severe depression and withdrawal.

Complete rejection of child and/or family.

Inability to function in family role.

Rivalrous, competitive, destructive and abusive to child.

Abetting child's acting-out of unacceptable sexual or aggressive impulses for vicarious reasons.

Complete inability to socialize or work (learning, etc.).

Psychoses.

Perpetuation of incapacitating infantilism in the pre-adolescent.

Panic reactions to acceptable standards of sexual behavior, social activity and assertiveness.

Compulsive, obsessive or psychotic behavior.

APPENDIX C

THE DIAGNOSTIC NOMENCLATURE:
List of Mental Disorders and Their Code Numbers

I. MENTAL RETARDATION (310-315)

310	Borderline mental retardation
311	Mild mental retardation
312	Moderate mental retardation
313	Severe mental retardation
314	Profound mental retardation
315	Unspecified mental retardation

The fourth-digit sub-divisions cited below should be used with each of the above categories. The associated physical condition should be specified as an additional diagnosis when known.

.0	Following infection or intoxication
.1	Following trauma or physical agent
.2	With disorders of metabolism, growth or nutrition
.3	Associated with gross brain disease (postnatal)
.4	Associated with diseases and conditions due to (unknown) prenatal influence
.5	With chromosomal abnormality
.6	Associated with prematurity
.7	Following major psychiatric disorder
.8	With psychosocial (environmental) deprivation
.9	With other [and unspecified] condition

II. ORGANIC BRAIN SYNDROMES
(Disorders Caused by or Associated With Impairment of Brain Tissue Function). In the categories under IIA and IIB, the associated physical condition should be specified when known.

II-A. PSYCHOSES ASSOCIATED WITH ORGANIC BRAIN SYNDROMES (290-294)

290	Senile and pre-senile dementia
.0	Senile dementia
.1	Pre-senile dementia

291	Alcoholic psychosis
.0	Delirium tremens
.1	Korsakov's psychosis (alcoholic)
.2	Other alcoholic hallucinosis
.3	Alcohol paranoid state (Alcoholic paranoia)
.4*	Acute alcohol intoxication*
.5*	Alcoholic deterioration*
.6*	Pathological intoxiation*
.9	Other/and unspecified/alcoholic psychosis

292	Psychosis associated with intracranial infection
.0	Psychosis with general paralysis
.1	Psychosis with other syphilis of central nervous system
.2	Psychosis with epidemic encephalitis
.3	Psychosis with other and unspecified encephalitis
.9	Psychosis with other/and unspecified/intracranial infection

293	Psychosis associated with other cerebral condition
.0	Psychosis with cerebral arteriosclerosis
.1	Psychosis with other cerebrovascular disturbance
.2	Psychosis with epilepsy
.3	Psychosis with intracranial neoplasm
.4	Psychosis with degenerative disease of the central nervous system
.5	Psychosis with brain trauma
.9	Psychosis with other/and unspecified/cerebral condition

294	Psychosis associated with other physical condition
.0	Psychosis with endocrine disorder
.1	Psychosis with metabolic or nutritional disorder
.2	Psychosis with systemic infection
.3	Psychosis with drug or poison intoxication (other than alcohol)
.4	Psychosis with childbirth
.8	Psychosis with other and undiagnosed physical condition
/.9	Psychosis with unspecified physical condition/

II-B. NONPSYCHOTIC ORGANIC BRAIN SYNDROMES (309)

309	Nonpsychotic organic brain syndromes (Mental disorders not specified as psychotic associated with physical conditions)
.0	Nonpsychotic OBS with intracranial infection
/.1	Nonpsychotic OBS with drug, poison, or systemic intoxication/
.13*	Nonpsychotic OBS with alcohol* (simple drunkenness)
.14*	Nonpsychotic OBS with other drug, poison, or systemic intoxication*
.2	Nonpsychotic OBS with brain trauma
.3	Nonpsychotic OBS with circulatory disturbance
.4	Nonpsychotic OBS with epilepsy
.5	Nonpsychotic OBS with disturbance of metabolism, growth or nutrition
.6	Nonpsychotic OBS with senile or pre-senile brain disease

.7   Nonpsychotic OBS with degenerative disease of central nervous system
.9   Nonpsychotic OBS with other/and unspecified/physical condition
 /.91* Acute brain syndrome, not otherwise specified*/
 /.92* Chronic brain syndrome, not otherwise specified*/

III. PSYCHOSES NOT ATTRIBUTED TO PHYSICAL CONDITIONS LISTED PREVIOUSLY (295-298)

295 Schizophrenia
.0 Schizophrenia, simple type
.1 Schizophrenia, hebephrenic type
.2 Schizophrenia, catatonic type
 .23* Schizophrenia, catatonic type, excited*
 .24* Schizophrenia, catatonic type, withdrawn*
.3 Schizophrenia, paranoid type
.4 Acute schizophrenic episode
.5 Schizophrenia, latent type
.6 Schizophrenia, residual type
.7 Schizophrenia, schizo-affective type
 .73* Schizophrenia, schizo-affective type, excited*
 .74* Schizophrenia, schizo-affective type, depressed*
.8* Schizophrenia, childhood type*
.90* Schizophrenia, chronic undifferentiated type*
.99* Schizophrenia, other/and unspecified/types*

296 Major affective disorders (Affective psychoses)
.0 Involutional melancholia
.1 Manic-depressive illness, manic type (Manic-depressive psychosis, manic type)
.2 Manic-depressive illness, depressed type (Manic-depressive psychosis, depressed type)
.3 Manic-depressive illness, circular type (Manic-depressive psychosis, circular type)
 .33* Manic-depressive illness, circular type, manic*
 .34* Manic-depressive illness, circular type, depressed*
.8 Other major affective disorder (Affective psychoses, other)
/.9 Unspecified major affective disorder/
  /Affective disorder not otherwise specified/
  /Manic-depressive illness not otherwise specified/

297 Paranoid states
.0 Paranoia
.1 Involutional paranoid state (Involutional paraphrenia)
.9 Other paranoid state

298 Other psychoses
.0 Psychotic depressive reaction (Reactive depressive psychosis)
/.1 Reactive excitation/
/.2 Reactive confusion/
  /Acute or subacute confusional state/
/.3 Acute paranoid reaction/
/.9 Reactive psychosis, unspecified/

/299   Unspecified psychosis/
              /Dementia, insanity or psychosis not otherwise specified/

IV. NEUROSES (300)

300	Neuroses
.0	Anxiety neurosis
.1	Hysterical neurosis
.13*	Hysterical neurosis, conversion type*
.14*	Hysterical neurosis, dissociative type*
.2	Phobic neurosis
.3	Obsessive compulsive neurosis
.4	Depressive neurosis
.5	Neurasthenic neurosis (Neurasthenia)
.6	Depersonalization neurosis (Depersonalization syndrome)
.7	Hypochondriacal neurosis
.8	Other neurosis
/.9	Unspecified neurosis/

V. PERSONALITY DISORDERS AND CERTAIN OTHER NONPSYCHOTIC MENTAL DISORDERS (301-304)

301	Personality disorders
.0	Paranoid personality
.1	Cyclothymic personality ((Affective personality))
.2	Schizoid personality
.3	Explosive personality
.4	Obsessive compulsive personality ((Anankastic personality))
.5	Hysterical personality
.6	Asthenic personality
.7	Antisocial personality
.81*	Passive-aggressive personality*
.82*	Inadequate personality*
.89*	Other personality disorders of specified types*
/.9	Unspecified personality disorder/

302	Sexual deviations
.0	Homosexuality
.1	Fetishism
.2	Pedophilia
.3	Transvestitism
.4	Exhibitionism
.5*	Voyeurism*
.6*	Sadism*
.7*	Masochism*
.8	Other sexual deviation
/.9	Unspecified sexual deviation/

303	Alcoholism
.0	Episodic excessive drinking
.1	Habitual excessive drinking
.2	Alcohol addiction
.9	Other/and unspecified/alcoholism

304	Drug dependence
.0	Drug dependence, opium, opium alkaloids and their derivatives
.1	Drug dependence, synthetic analgesics with morphine-like effects
.2	Drug dependence, barbiturates
.3	Drug dependence, other hypnotics and sedatives or "tranquilizers"
.4	Drug dependence, cocaine
.5	Drug dependence, Cannabis sativa (hashish, marijuana)
.6	Drug dependence, other psycho-stimulants
.7	Drug dependence, hallucinogens
.8	Other drug dependence
/.9	Unspecified drug dependence/

VI. PSYCHOPHYSIOLOGIC DISORDERS (305)

305	Psychophysiologic disorders ((Physical disorders of presumably psychogenic origin))
.0	Psychophysiologic skin disorder
.1	Psychophysiologic musculoskeletal disorder
.2	Psychophysiologic respiratory disorder
.3	Psychophysiologic cardiovascular disorder
.4	Psychophysiologic hemic and lymphatic disorder
.5	Psychophysiologic gastro-intestinal disorder
.6	Psychophysiologic genito-urinary disorder
.7	Psychophysiologic endocrine disorder
.8	Psychophysiologic disorder of organ of special sense
.9	Psychophysiologic disorder of other type

VII. SPECIAL SYMPTOMS (306)

306	Special symptoms not elsewhere classified
.0	Speech disturbance
.1	Specific learning disturbance
.2	Tic
.3	Other psychomotor disorder
.4	Disorders of sleep
.5	Feeding disturbance
.6	Enuresis
.7	Encopresis
.8	Cephalalgia
.9	Other special symptom

VIII. TRANSIENT SITUATIONAL DISTURBANCES (307)

307*	Transient situational disturbances[1]
.0*	Adjustment reaction of infancy*
.1*	Adjustment reaction of childhood*
.2*	Adjustment reaction of adolescence*
.3*	Adjustment reaction of adult life*
.4*	Adjustment reaction of late life*

IX. BEHAVIOR DISORDERS OF CHILDHOOD AND ADOLESCENCE (308)

308	Behavior disorders of childhood and adolescence[2] ((Behavior disorders of childhood))
.0*	Hyperkinetic reaction of childhood (or adolescence)*
.1*	Withdrawing reaction of childhood (or adolescence)*
.2*	Overanxious reaction of childhood (or adolescence)*
.3*	Runaway reaction of childhood (or adolescence)*
.4*	Unsocialized aggressive reaction of childhood (or adolescence)*
.5*	Group delinquent reaction of childhood (or adolescence)*
.9*	Other reaction of childhood (or adolescence)*

X. CONDITIONS WITHOUT MANIFEST PSYCHIATRIC DISORDER AND NONSPECIFIC CONDITIONS (316*-318*)[+]

316*++	Social maladjustments without manifest psychiatric disorder
.0*	Marital maladjustment*
.1*	Social maladjustment*
.2*	Occupational maladjustment*
.3*	Dyssocial behavior*
.9*	Other social maladjustment*

317*	Nonspecific conditions*

318*	No mental disorder*

XI. NONDIAGNOSTIC TERMS FOR ADMINISTRATIVE USE (319*)[+]

319*	Nondiagnostic terms for administrative use*
.1*	Boarder*
.2*	Experiment only*
.9*	Other*

[1] The terms included under DSM-11 Category 307*, "Transient situational disturbances", differ from those in Category 307 of the ICD. DSM-11 Category 307*, "Transient situational disturbances", contains adjustment reactions of infancy (307.0*), childhood (307.1*), adolescence (307.2*), adult life (307.3*), and late life (307.4*). ICD Category 307, "Transient situational disturbances", includes only the adjustment reactions of adolescence, adult life and late life. ICD 308, "Behavioral disorders of children", contains the reactions of infancy and childhood. These differences must be taken into account in preparing statistical tabulations to conform to ICD categories.

[2] The terms included under DSM-11 Category 308*, "Behavioral disorders of childhood and adolescence", differ from those in Category 308 of the ICD. DSM-11 Category 308* includes "Behavioral disorders of childhood and adolescence", whereas ICD Category 308 includes only "Behavioral disorders of childhood". DSM-11 Category 308* does not include "Adjustment reactions of infancy and childhood", whereas ICD Category 308 does. In the DSM-11 classification, "Adjustment reactions of infancy and

childhood" are allocated to 307* (Transitional situational disturbances). These differences should be taken into account in preparing statistical tabulations to conform to the ICD categories.

+ The terms included in this category would normally be listed in that section of ICD-8 that deals with "Special conditions and examinations without sickness". They are included here to permit coding of some additional conditions that are encountered in psychiatric clinical settings in the United States. This has been done by using several unassigned code numbers at the end of Section 5 of the ICD.

++ This diagnosis corresponds to the category *Y13, Social maladjustment without manifest psychiatric disorder in ICDA.

The brackets indicate categories in The International Classification of Diseases, Eighth Revision, World Health Organization, 1968, used in the United States only by record librarians.

Double parentheses indicate ICD-8 terms equivalent to United States terms.

Asterisks indicate categories added to the ICD-8 for use only in the United States.

APPENDIX D

MENTAL STATUS EXAMINATION FOR PSYCHIATRIC PATIENTS*

The Mental Status: The Mental Status Examination is a way of organizing observational data. The mental condition of the patient can be observed during the history taking, and only a few areas may require additional questioning. As with the history, the system of recording varies, but the purpose of the record is to describe the patient and his mental functioning as he appears to the interviewer and as he describes himself. In the mental status examination are observations of the patient. The inferences concerning these observations should be placed in the diagnostic formulation. The headings under which information is recorded in the mental examination are descriptive areas of mental functioning the examiner wishes to explore.

1. Appearance, Attitude and Activity: During the interview, the examiner should observe the following to be recorded later:

    a. The patient's general physical appearance; his state of health and estimated age; his manner; his characteristic facial expression and mobility (placid, vacant, bewildered, apprehensive, alert, eager); and the appropriateness, neatness and manner of dress and grooming.

* Adapted from Merrill T. Eaton, Jr., and Margaret H. Peterson, Psychiatry, Second Edition, Medical Outline Series. New York: Medical Examination Publishing Company, 1969.

b. The patient's reaction to the examiner and the examination, taking into account the circumstances of the interview, (cooperative, friendly, courteous, ingratiating, over-eager, hostile, sullen, evasive, etc.).

c. The character and amount of motor activity, any indications of restlessness or anxiety, and the presence of mannerisms or tics; abnormalities of motor response such as sustained hyperactivity, extreme slowness or retardation, echopraxia (the pathological repetition of movements made by others) or cerea flexibilitas (the "waxy flexibility" of the catatonic states in which the patient will maintain unnatural postures in which he has been placed).

2. Thought Processes: As the patient talks, the examiner should note the following:

a. The degree of productivity and the patient's spontaneity.

b. Coherence and continuity of thought and the patient's ability to reach goal ideas, the relevance of his productions and the character of his associations (whether the connection between one expressed thought and the following one is appropriate and readily seen or peculiar and sometimes obscure).

c. The speed of reaction and manner of answering direct questions.

d. The presence of abnormalities such as:

(1) Blocking - a sudden interruption of thought or speech, usually resulting from unconscious emotional factors.

(2) Mutism - refusal to speak, often seen in psychosis.

(3) Echolalia - meaningless repetition of words spoken by the examiner.

(4) Neologisms - new words formed to express symbolic or condensed ideas. Neologisms must be differentiated from technical words, slang and other words which may not be familiar to the examiner.

(5) Flight of ideas - skipping from one idea to another in a fragmented rapid fashion in response to chance stimuli, to be distinguished from rambling in which the person reaches goal ideas by seemingly aimless routes, and looseness of association in which the connection between thoughts is obscure.

(6) Perseveration - involuntary repetition of the answer to a previous question in response to new questions.

3. Thought Content: In the course of the interview, patients may tell of areas of preoccupation spontaneously, but if they do not, the ex-

aminer may need to question. Some patients who are troubled by unwanted recurring thoughts (obsessions) or who have unreasonable baseless fears (phobias) are eager to reveal them to the examiner, others may be reluctant. If the patient's educational level is such that he could reasonably be expected to be familiar with the terms hallucinations (false sensory perceptions without external stimulus) and delusions (persistent false beliefs not in keeping with the person's culture or education) he may be asked directly about them. If he hesitates, or appears not to understand, the examiner can rephrase his question to ask about experiences which the patient believes to be strange or that others may think of as strange. He may ask if the patient has seen or heard things which were not real or that others believe are not real. He may have to question about tendencies to misinterpret events or conversations, and about the patient's feeling of being singled out, watched or the subject of talk (ideas of reference). If the patient says that he hears voices or assumes a listening attitude so that the examiner could infer he is hearing voices, the examiner should not say "What are the voices saying to you?" since the question implies that the examiner believes that the hallucination is real.

4. Emotional State: Under this heading, the examiner should record the emotional components or feeling tone of the ideas expressed (the affect) and the more pervasive overall feeling tone (the mood). This is inferred from the interview behavior and the patient's statements It is not always necessary or appropriate to make inquiry. The examiner's empathic responses to the patient may give clues to the appropriateness of the affect or the character of the prevailing mood. Genuine sadness or anxiety tend to generate corresponding feelings in the observer. The examiner should assess the following:

a. Appropriateness of the emotions shown to the circumstances of the interview and the ideas being expressed.

b. Range of emotional expression including superficiality, apathy, diminution or exaggeration of response. This may include varying degrees of disturbance of affect such as a narrowed range of response, blunting, or flatness.

c. The presence of lability, and whether it is in response to major and minor shifts in content or occurs without stimulus.

d. Pervasive elation, undue optimism, or euphoria (a sense of well-being, noted if exaggerated or inappropriate) and the grandiosity sometimes accompanying these feelings.

e. Depression, or a prevailing attitude of pessimism. It should be noted if the depression is constant or if it lifts with appropriate stimulation. The concomitant feelings which may be expected with depression would include hopelessness, helplessness and guilt. If depression is present and the patient does not make spontaneous reference to suicide, the examiner should endeavor to bring out the patient's thoughts about self-destruction. For example, he might say, "Along with your feelings of despondency, (hopelessness, sadness) to what extent have you been troubled with thoughts of suicide"?

5. Sensorium and Intelligence: In the course of history taking, many aspects of the mental functioning can be observed. Detailed investigation of the sensorium or of the intelligence level may be necessary when there is a suggestion of confusion, intellectual deficit, or neurological disease. The examiner needs to explain the purpose of his line of questioning. In some instances, evaluation of the recent and remote memory or of recall can be incorporated into the neurological examination. The following areas should be evaluated:

a. Orientation - If the patient has made his way to the interview unaccompanied and has arrived at the appointed hour on the correct day, he can be assumed to be oriented as to time, place and person. If there is a reasonable doubt about this, he may be asked to tell where he is (what place, city, state) and the time of day, day of the week, the month or year.

b. Memory - The patient's ability to give a consistent account of his present illness and his past history may make specific tests for memory unnecessary. If testing is indicated, the examiner should assess the patient's recent and remote memory, his retention and immediate recall and his recall after a delay. Items of general information may be used in testing memory. For example, the examiner may ask about recent headline news, the number of weeks in a year, and historical items. To test recall, after a delay he may ask the patient to remember a word or number to be asked for later in the interview.

c. Arithmetic ability - Rote memory and auditory memory as well as arithmetic ability may be checked by asking the patient to repeat a series of digits, and by giving him simple problems and calculations. The ability to maintain a set may also be tested by asking him to do serial additions and subtractions.

d. Conceptual, concrete and abstract thinking - Evidence from the history may again be sufficient, but the examiner may wish to ask the patient to interpret several proverbs as "A bird in the hand is worth two in the bush", "Look before you leap", etc.

e. Intelligence level and special abilities - The patient's educational, occupational and attainment levels can help the interviewer assess these areas. Vocabulary can be a useful guide, but too much significance can be placed on this and on cultural differences. However, from the information of the history and the patient's manner of answering questions, the interviewer can often estimate the patient's basic intelligence level and the degree of impairment by the illness. The examiner may ask the patient to read stories, sentences or paragraphs to test reading ability, pronunciation, and comprehension. Vocabulary can be checked by asking for word definitions or synonyms. Questions on items of general information may be more appropriate here than in tests for memory and may be more extensive. If, after doing some general tests of intelligence and attempting to assess the patient's ability from his interview behavior, reasonable doubts about the patient's general level of intelligence or the possibility of deterioration arise, psychological testing may be requested.

f. Judgment - If the patient's judgment cannot be assessed from his account of past decisions and how they were reached, and if information about his ability to tolerate stress, defer pleasure and control his impulses is insufficient, several hypothetical situations may be offered for the patient to evaluate. He may ask what the patient would do if lost in a forest, in a strange city, or what his course of action would be if he found a stamped addressed letter on the street. Some measure of judgment may be found in the appropriateness of the patient's interview behavior. Example: he "spoils the response" of giving the correct answer, by sneering or adding a comment as "That's what you wanted me to say, isn't it?"

g. Insight - Some evaluation should be made of the patient's understanding of his own personality, and of his awareness of the nature of his problems (i.e., does he know that he is sick and how accurately does he estimate the degree of his disability?) The examiner should assess the candidness of the patient's estimate, noting if the patient minimizes or dramatizes his plight.

After recording the observations of the Mental Examination, the interviewer interprets the findings, grouping related findings into known clinical descriptions to establish the diagnosis, estimate the prognosis, and plan indicated treatment.

APPENDIX E

A PATIENT'S BILL OF RIGHTS[1]

The American Hospital Association presents a Patient's Bill of Rights with the expectation that observance of these rights will contribute to more effective patient care and greater satisfaction for the patient, his physician, and the hospital organization. Further, the Association presents these rights in the expectation that they will be supported by the hospital on behalf of its patients, as an integral part of the healing process. It is recognized that a personal relationship between the physician and the patient is essential for the provision of proper medical care. The traditional physician-patient relationship takes on a new dimension when care is rendered within an organizational structure. Legal precedent has established that the institution itself has a responsibility to the patient. It is in recognition of these factors that these rights are affirmed.

1. The patient has the right to considerate respectful care.

2. The patient has the right to obtain from his physician complete current information concerning his diagnosis, treatment, and prognosis in terms the patient can be reasonably expected to understand. When it is not medically advisable to give such information to the patient, the information should be made available to an appropriate

person in his behalf. He has the right to know by name the physician responsible for coordinating his care.

3. The patient has the right to receive from his physician information necessary to give informed consent prior to the start of any procedure and/or treatment. Except in emergencies, such information for informed consent should include but not necessarily be limited to the specific procedure and/or treatment, the medically significant risks involved, and the probable duration of incapacitation. Where medically significant alternatives for care or treatment exist, or when the patient requests information concerning medical alternatives, the patient has the right to such information. The patient also has the right to know the name of the person responsible for the procedures and/or treatment.

4. The patient has the right to refuse treatment to the extent permitted by law, and to be informed of the medical consequences of his action.

5. The patient has the right to every consideration of his privacy concerning his own medical care program. Case discussion, consultation, examination, and treatment are confidential and should be conducted discreetly. Those not directly involved in his care must have the permission of the patient to be present.

6. The patient has the right to expect that all communications and records pertaining to his care should be treated as confidential.

7. The patient has the right to expect that within its capacity, a hospital must make reasonable response to the request of a patient for services. The hospital must provide evaluation, service, and/or referral as indicated by the urgency of the case. When medically permissible a patient may be transferred to another facility only after he has received complete information and explanation concerning the needs for and alternatives to such a transfer. The institution to which the patient is to be transferred must first have accepted the patient for transfer.

8. The patient has the right to obtain information as to any relationship of his hospital to other health care and educational institutions insofar as his care is concerned. The patient has the right to obtain information as to the existence of any professional relationships among individuals, by name, who are treating him.

9. The patient has the right to be advised if the hospital proposes to engage in or perform human experimentation affecting his care or treatment. The patient has the right to refuse to participate in such research projects.

10. The patient has the right to expect reasonable continuity of care. He has the right to know in advance what appointment times and physicians are available and where. The patient has the right to expect that the hospital will provide a mechanism whereby he is informed by his physician or delegate of the physician of the patient's continuing health care requirements following discharge.

11. The patient has the right to examine and receive an explanation of his bill regardless of source of payment.

12. The patient has the right to know what hospital rules and regulations apply to his conduct as a patient.

No catalogue of rights can guarantee for the patient the kind of treatment he has a right to expect. A hospital has many functions to perform including the prevention and treatment of disease, the education of both health professionals and patients, and the conduct of clinical research. And these activities must be conducted with an overriding concern for the patient, and, above all, the recognition of his dignity as a human being. Success in achieving this recognition assures success in the defense of the rights of the patient.

[1] The Board of Trustees of the American Hospital Association on November 17, 1972, affirmed a statement on a patient's bill of rights which has met with considerable interest in the health care field. This is the complete statement. (Reprinted with the permission of the American Hospital Association.)

APPENDIX F

STANDARDS: PSYCHIATRIC-MENTAL HEALTH NURSING PRACTICE[1]

STANDARD I: Data are collected through pertinent clinical observations based on knowledge of the arts and sciences, with particular emphasis upon psychosocial and biophysical sciences.

Rationale: Clinical observation is a prerequisite to realistic assessment of a client's needs and for the formulation of appropriate intervention. Observations can be facilitated through knowledge derived from a broad general education. In addition, scholarship acquired in the study of psychosocial and biophysical sciences fosters acuity of perception and alerts the nurse to psychologic, cultural, social and other relevant clinical data.

Assessment Factors

1. Data collecting activities involve observation, analysis and interpretation of behavior patterns of clients which indicate a need for growth promoting relationships.
2. Data collecting activities involve identification of significant areas in which clinical data are needed.
3. Data collecting activities involve utilization of knowledge derived from appropriate sources to gain a comprehensive grasp of the client's experience.
4. Data collecting activities involve inferences drawn from observations which contribute to a formulation of therapeutic intervention.
5. Data collecting activities involve inferences and treatment observations which are shared and validated with appropriate others.

STANDARD II: Clients are involved in the assessment, planning, implementation and evaluation of their nursing care program to the fullest extent of their capabilities.

Rationale: To a very large degree, the therapeutic process is a learning process. The same principle that applies to learning also applies to therapy; that is, the learner or client must be an active participant in the process. The ability to participate in such a process will vary from person to person and, at times, even within the same person. The word "therapy" is used here in its broadest sense; that is, any behavior or planned activity that promotes growth and well-being. Thus, "nursing care program" and "nursing therapy" are interchangeably used, although it is recognized that many other forms of therapy exist.

Assessment Factors

1. Client's capabilities to participate at any given time are assessed, always keeping in mind the ultimate goals mutually determined by the client and nurse.
2. Plans for achieving and re-examining the goals are developed with the client, making whatever readjustments are necessary to progress toward them.
3. Problems are identified in collaboration with the client to determine needs and to set goals.
4. Progress of clients toward mutual goal achievement is assessed.

STANDARD III: The problem-solving approach is utilized in developing nursing care plans.

Rationale: A nursing diagnosis is based on pertinent theories of human behavior. It is used to plan therapeutic intervention taking into consideration the characteristics and capacities of the individual and his environment in order to maximize the treatment program for the client.

Assessment Factors

1. The individual's reaction to the environment is observed and assessed.
2. Themes and patterns of the behavior are observed and assessed.
3. Nursing care plans are used as a guide to nursing intervention.
4. Nursing care plans are interpreted to professional and nonprofessional persons giving care.
5. Observations and reports of others are incorporated in the nursing care plans.
6. Nursing care plans are designed, implemented and reviewed systematically by the nursing staff.

STANDARD IV: Individuals, families and community groups are assisted to achieve satisfying and productive patterns of living through health teaching.

Rationale: Health teaching is an essential part of a nurse's role in work with those who have mental health problems. Every interaction can be utilized as a teaching-learning situation. Formal and informal teaching methods can be used in working with individuals, families, the community and other personnel. Emphasis is on understanding mental health problems as well as on developing ways of coping with them.

Assessment Factors

1. The needs of individual, family and community groups for health teaching are identified and appropriate techniques are used in meeting these needs.
2. The principles of learning and teaching are employed.
3. The basic principles of physical and mental health and interpersonal and social skills are taught.
4. Experiential learning opportunities are made available.
5. Opporunities with community groups to further their knowledge and understanding of mental health problems are identified.

STANDARD V: The activities of daily living are utilized in a goal directed way in work with clients.

Rationale: A major portion of one's daily life is spent in some form of activity related to health and well-being. An individual's developmental and intellectual level, emotional state and physical limitations may be reflected in these activities. Therefore, nursing has a unique opportunity to assess and intervene in these processes in order to encourage constructive changes in the client's behavior so that each person may realize his full potential for growth.

Assessment Factors

1. An appraisal is made of the client's capacities to participate in activities of daily living based on needs, strengths and levels of functioning.
2. Clients are encouraged toward independence and self-direction by various skills such as motivating, limit setting, persuading, guiding and comforting.
3. Each person's rights are appreciated and respected.
4. Methods of cummunicating are devised which assure consistency in approach.

STANDARD VI: Knowledge of somatic therapies and related clinical skills are utilized in working with clients.

Rationale: Various treatment modalities may be needed by clients during the course of illness. Pertinent clinical observations and judgments are made concerning the effect of drugs and other treatments used in the therapeutic program.

Assessment Factors

1. Pertinent reactions to somatic therapies are observed and interpreted in terms of the underlying principles of each therapy.
2. A patient's responses are observed and reported.

3. The effectiveness of somatic therapies is judged and subsequent recommendations for changes in the treatment plan are made.
4. The safety and emotional support of client's receiving therapies is provided.
5. Opportunities are provided for clients and families to discuss, question and explore their feelings and concerns about past, current or projected use of somatic therapies.

STANDARD VII: The environment is structured to establish and maintain a therapeutic milieu.

Rationale: Any environment is composed of both human and nonhuman resources which may work for or against the person's well-being. The nurse works with people in a variety of environmental settings, e.g., hospital, home, etc. The milieu is structured and/or altered so that it serves the client's best interests as an inherent part of the overall therapeutic plan.

Assessment Factors

1. The effects of environmental forces on individuals are observed, analyzed and interpreted.
2. Psychological, physiological, social, economical and cultural concepts are understood and utilized in developing and maintaining a therapeutic milieu.
3. Communications within the environment are congruent with therapeutic goals.
4. All available resourses in the environment are utilized when appropriate in the therapeutic efforts.
5. Nursing participation and its effectiveness in establishing and maintaining a therapeutic milieu are evaluated.

STANDARD VIII: Nursing participates with interdisciplinary teams in assessing, planning, implementing and evaluating programs and other mental health activities.

Rationale: In addition to the nurse, the number and variety of people working with clients in the mental health field today make it imperative that efforts be coordinated to provide the best total program. Communication, planning, problem-solving and evaluation are required of all those who work with a particular client or program.

Assessment Factors

1. Specific knowledge, skills and activities are identified and articulated so these may be coordinated with the contributions of others working with a client or a program.
2. The value of nursing and team member contributions are recognized and respected.
3. Consultation with other team members is utilized as needed.
4. Nursing participates in the formulating of overall goals, plans and decisions.
5. Skills are developed in small group process for maximum team effectiveness.

STANDARD IX: Psychotherapeutic interventions are used to assist clients to achieve their maximum development.

Rationale: People with mental health problems fashion many of their patterns of living and relating to others on a psychopathologic basis. In order to help clients achieve better adaption and improved health, a nurse assists them to identify that which is useful and that which is not useful in their modes of living and relating. Alternatives available to them are identified.

Assessment Factors

1. Useful patterns and themes in the client's interactions with others are re-enforced.
2. Clients are assisted to identify, test out and evaluate more constructive alternatives to unsatisfactory patterns of living.
3. Principles of communication, problem-solving, interviewing and crisis intervention are employed in carrying through psychotherapeutic intervention.
4. Knowledge of psychopathology and its healthy adaptive counterparts are used in planning and implementing programs of care.
5. Limits are set on behavior that is destructive to self or others with the ultimate goal of assisting clients to develop their own internal controls and more constructive ways of dealing with feelings.
6. Crisis intervention is used to reduce panic of disturbed patients.
7. Long-term psychotherapeutic relationships with clients are undertaken.
8. Colleagues are utilized in evaluating the progress of the psychotherapeutic relationships and in formulating modification of intervention techniques.
9. Nursing participation in the therapeutic relationship is evaluated and modified as necessary.

STANDARD X: The practice of individual, group or family psychotherapy requires appropriate preparation and recognition of accountability for the practice.

Rationale: Acceptance of the role of therapist entails primary responsibility for the treatment of clients and entrance into a contractual agreement. This contract includes a commitment to see a client through the problem he presents or, if this becomes impossible, to assist him in finding other appropriate assistance. It also includes an explicit definition of the relationship, the respective roles of each person in the relationship, and what can realistically be expected of each person.

Assessment Factors

1. The potential of the nurse to function as a primary therapist is evaluated.
2. The accountability for practicing psychotherapy is recognized and accepted.

3. Knowledge of growth and development, psychopathology, psycho-social systems and small group and family dynamics is utilized in the therapeutic process.
4. The terms of the contract between the nurse and the client, including the structure of time, place, fees, etc., that may be involved, are made explicitly clear.
5. Supervision or consultation is sought whenever indicated and other learning opportunities are used to further develop knowledge and skills.
6. The effectiveness of the work with an individual, family or group is routinely assessed.

STANDARD XI: Nursing participates with other members of the community in planning and implementing mental health services that include the broad continuum of promotion of mental health, prevention of mental illness, treatment and rehabilitation.

Rationale: In our contemporary society, the high incidence of mental illness and mental retardation requires increased effort to devise more effective treatment and prevention programs. There is a need for nursing to participate in programs that strengthen the existing health potential of all members of society. In this effort, cooperation and collaboration by all community agencies becomes imperative. Such concepts as early intervention and continuity of care are essential in planning to meet the mental health needs of the community. The nurse uses organizational, advisory or consultative skills to facilitate the development and implementation of mental health services.

Assessment Factors

1. Knowledge of community and group dynamics is used to understand the structure and function of the community system.
2. Current social issues that influence the nature of mental health problems in the community are recognized.
3. High risk population groups in the community are delineated and gaps in community services are identified.
4. Community members are encouraged to become active in assessing community mental health needs and planning programs to meet these needs.
5. The strength and capacities of individuals, families and the community are assessed in order to promote and increase the health potential of all.
6. Consultative skills are used to facilitate the development and implementation of mental health services.
7. The needs of the community are brought to the attention of appropriate individuals and groups, including legislative bodies and regional and state planning boards.
8. The mental health services of the agency are interpreted to others in the community. There is collaboration with the staff of other agencies to insure continuity of service for patients and families.
9. Community resources are used appropriately.

10. Nursing participates with other professional and nonprofessional members of the community in the planning, implementation and evaluation of mental health services.

STANDARD XII: Learning experiences are provided for other nursing care personnel through leadership, supervision and teaching.

Rationale: As leader of the nursing team, the nurse is responsible for the team's activities, and must be able to teach, supervise and evaluate the performance of nursing care personnel. The focus is on the continuing development of each member of the team.

Assessment Factors

1. Leadership roles and responsibilities are accepted.
2. Team members are encouraged to identify strengths and abilities. A climate is provided for the continuing self-development of each member.
3. A role model in giving direct nursing care is provided for the team.
4. The supervisory role is used as a tool for improving nursing care.
5. The client's needs, as well as the abilities of each member of the nursing team, are evaluated and assignments are based on these evaluations.

STANDARD XIII: Responsibility is assumed for continuing educational and professional development and contributions are made to the professional growth of others.

Rationale: The scientific, cultural and social changes characterizing our contemporary society require the nurse to be committed to the ongoing pursuit of knowledge which will enhance professional growth.

Assessment Factors

1. There is evidence of study of one's nursing practice to increase both understanding and skill.
2. There is evidence of participation in in-service meetings and educational programs either as an attendee or as a teacher.
3. There is evidence of attendance at conventions, institutes, workshops, symposia and other professionally oriented meetings and/or other ways to increase formal education.
4. There is evidence of systematic efforts to increase understanding of psychodynamics, psychopathology and avenues of psychotherapeutic intervention.
5. There is evidence of cognizance of developments in relevant fields and utilization of this knowledge.
6. There is evidence of assisting others to identify areas of educational needs.
7. There is evidence of sharing appropriate clinical observations and interpretations with professionals and other groups.

STANDARD XIV: Contributions to nursing and the mental health field are made through innovations in theory and practice and participation in research.

Rationale: Each professional has responsibility for the continuing development and refinement of knowledge in the mental health field through research and experimentation with new and creative approaches to practice.

Assessment Factors

1. Studies are developed, implemented and evaluated.
2. Responsible standards of research are used in investigative endeavors.
3. Nursing practice is approached with an inquiring and open mind.
4. The pertinent and responsible research of others is supported.
5. Expert consultation and/or supervision is sought as required.
6. The ability to discriminate those findings which are pertinent to the advancement of nursing practice is demonstrated.
7. Innovations in theory, practice and research findings are made available through presentations and/or publications.

[1] American Nurses' Association, 1973

EXERCISES

There are no right answers here. The exercises are for your own growth, your own private thoughts. If you would like to discuss your answers, contact the author, in care of the publisher.

1. Explain the institution of marriage using Freud's theory; using Piaget's theory.

2. A four- or five-year-old child on the unit often refuses to eat. How would your nursing interventions differ if you were philosophically Freudian? Eriksonian? Sullivanian? Piagetian? Rogerian?

3. A sociopathic young man is in therapy. How might his behavior differ in individual therapy? Reality therapy? Group therapy?

4. How might the "nursing" intervention differ in the above situation - before and after, not during, therapy?

5. Psychodynamics is based on unconscious motivation and Freudian developmental theory. In what other ways could you explain depression or elation?

6. For many years schizophrenia has been viewed as resulting from a morbid family relationship. How would you intervene in such a malfunctioning family structure? Do you agree with the "family" explanation?

7. Drug addiction is occurring more frequently in all age groups. How would your approach and nursing interventions differ with a ten-year-old boy? 16-year-old girl? 25-year-old woman? 40-year-old man? 85-year-old man?

8. An alcoholic rarely does well in analytic or in individual therapy; he may be able to alter his behavior in group therapy, sometimes in family therapy. How can you account for this difference? How would this behavior affect your nursing interventions with the alcoholic?

9. A nurse needs to know her actual feelings about various behaviors, in order to help patients have positive experiences. If she does not realize how she feels, or refuses to face her feelings, she can give patients negative nongrowth producing experiences.
   a. How do you feel about alcoholics? Drug addicts? Homosexuals? Sociopaths?
   b. Do you become angry when others are aggressive towards you? Superior towards you? Reject you?
   c. Can you be calm in a hostile group? Do you function better on a one-to-one relationship? Or in a larger group? Or in a small group?
   d. Are you easily manipulated? Are you able to manipulate others?
   e. Several types of behaviors, developmental stages, and age groups have been discussed in this book. To work with, which ones appeal to you the most? The least?

Homeostasis, 28, 166-168
Homosexual
  attitudes towards, 14, 50, 66
  intervention, 108-109
  Oedipal resolution, 50, 66,
        106-108
  panic, 66
  paranoid, 94-95
  psychodynamics, 105, 106-108
Hospital Picture Test, 151
Hospitalization
  avoidance of, 12, 176
  community mental health
        centers and, 185
  custodial care, 8
  day, 190-191
  emergency, 190-191
  evening, 191
  functions, 186
  general, 186
  history, 8-12
  mental illness and, 69, 185
  night, 191
  partial, 190-191, 194
  private, 186-187
  psychiatric teams, 189
  public, 186-187
  readmission, 67, 193
  ward meetings, 189
  weekend, 191
Hospitalized Child, 150-151
Hostile (see Behaviors)
How to Read a Person Like a
        Book, 38
Human Potential Movement,
        177
Humiliation, 83, 127, 143
Hydroxyzine (Atarax), 202
Hyperactivity, 69, 81, 84, 133
Hypertensive Crisis, 204-205
Hyperventilation, 61-62
Hypochondriasis, 61
Hypnosis, 210-211
Hypothesis, 43-44, 55, 70
Hysteria, 62
Hysterical Blindness, 62

Id
  binding, 167
  capitulation in neurosis, 81,
        87
  capitulation in psychoses, 81,
        87, 95, 99
  impulses, 22

structure, 22
Idealized Self, 43, 75, 181
Ideas, Flight of (see Flight)
Ideas of Reference, 94
Identification
  with the aggressor, 100
  group, 173
  imitation, 26, 118, 153-154
  of patient, 23, 163
  resolution, 50
Identity
  adolescent, 123-125
  basic need in reality therapy, 179
  crisis, 133
  gender, 51, 66, 102, 108-110, 117
  versus role diffusion, 183
  self concept and, 42-43, 51
  middle age, 133
Illusions, 102, 142-143
Imipramine (Tofranil), 203
Imitation, 26, 54, 118
Immigrants, 7
Implosive, 182
Impulse Control, 86, 101
Incest, 107
Incorporation, 95, 100, 106
Independent Functions of the Nurse,
        13-18
Induction, 166
Infantile, 65, 99
Inferences, 35, 42
Inferiority versus Industry, 53
Initiative versus Guilt, 53
"Inside-Outside" Body, 123
Insight, 36, 64, 66-67, 76, 140,
        149, 178-179
Insulin Shock, 9
Integration, 53, 54, 153
Interactions, 165-166, 173, 205-
        206
Interpersonal Relations in Nursing,
        10
Integrity versus Despair, 54
Interventions, Nursing
  adolescent, 127
  antisocial, 100-102
  anxious, 64-67
  autistic child, 117-118
  defined, 43, 58
  depressed, 75-78
  deviant, 108-110
  elated, 82-84
  interpersonal accuracy and, 42
  involutional, 135-137

Other Books of Interest

Psychiatric Community Mental Health Nursing Case Studies

by

MARGERY M. CHISHOLM, R.N., M.S., Ed.D.
GAIL G. HAMILTON, R.N., M.S.
CLARE O'CALLAGHAN, R.N., M.S.
CONSTANCE C. ROSENBERGER, R.N., M.S.
Boston University School of Nursing
Boston, Massachusetts

321 pages ● **1976** ● **$7.50**

A volume of 51 case histories which incorporate pertinent study questions based on the case material, fully detailed explanations of the answers, and selected references. Designed to increase the nurse's awareness of opportunities for preventive intervention, health teaching, and the formulation of treatment and rehabilitative plans. **(#391)**

Psychiatric-Mental Health Nursing Continuing Education Review

by

Dorothea R. Hays, R.N., M.S.
Eleanore G. Alesi, R.N., M.S.
Helen M. Arnold, R.N., M.S.
Barbara S. Joyce, R.N., M.A.
Elaine A. Pasquali, R.N., M.S.

198 pages ★ **1973** ★ **$7.00**

A review comprising 495 essay questions and detailed answers extensively referenced to current literature. Provides summaries of topics in new areas of special interest to nurses, psychiatric-mental health aides, and medical personnel in the field. **(#351)**

PSYCHIATRY
Medical Outline Series

Third Edition

By

MERRILL T. EATON, Jr., M.D.
Professor of Psychiatry
University of Nebraska College of Medicine
Omaha, Nebraska

MARGARET H. PETERSON, M.D.
Associate Clinical Professor of Psychiatry
University of California, Irvine
California College of Medicine
Irvine, California

JAMES A. DAVIS, M.D.
Associate Professor of Psychiatry
University of Nebraska College of Medicine
Omaha, Nebraska

510 Pages • **1976** • **$9.00**

A concise outline of Psychiatry, specifically designed to acquaint the student with basic concepts of disease and therapy. Divided into four major parts, this volume begins with a thorough presentation of basic concepts. Symptoms, diagnosis, prevention, and treatment are all clearly detailed within the context of each disorder. Part II presents various clinical entities. In Part III, the various treatment modalities are explained and the roles of different facilities are discussed. Part IV outlines psychiatry's relation to the law and its history. Selected references at the end of each chapter guide the reader to vital source material; a comprehensive index is also included.